P9-DGN-057

The Caregiving Dilemma

The Caregiving Dilemma

Work in an American Nursing Home

Nancy Foner

UNIVERSITY OF CALIFORNIA PRESS
Berkeley / Los Angeles / London

University of California Press
Berkeley and Los Angeles, California

University of California Press
London, England

Library of Congress Cataloging-in-Publication Data
Foner, Nancy, 1945–
The caregiving dilemma: work in an American nursing home/
Nancy Foner.
p. cm.
Includes bibliographical references and index.
ISBN 0–520–08359–8 (cloth)
1. Nursing home care. 2. Nurses' aides—Job stress.
3. Long-term care of the sick. I. Title.
RT120.L64F66 1994
362.1'6—dc20 93–27426
CIP

Printed in the United States of America

1 2 3 4 5 6 7 8 9

The paper used in this publication meets the minimum requirements of American National Standard for Information Sciences—Permanence of Paper for Printed Library Materials, ANSI Z39.48–1984 ♾

Contents

Preface

Any book about nursing homes is likely to touch a responsive chord. Most Americans approach the subject with a mixture of distress, sympathy, and, sometimes, political conviction based on what they have read, what they have seen in nursing homes they have visited, and what they fear, in the years ahead, for themselves and their loved ones. In a sense, nursing homes are too close for comfort. Unlike anthropological studies of distant lands and communities, an account of American nursing home life is likely to trigger personal reactions as many see, in the patients described, visions of themselves or their relatives now or in the future.

This study is an attempt by one outside observer to try to understand the dynamics, contradictions, and strains involved in caregiving in American nursing homes. At the center are the main caregivers, nursing aides. Obviously, nursing homes have been created to look after the frail elderly, yet in most facilities, there are nearly as many—sometimes more—employees as patients. Nursing home life is as much a story of the workers and their worlds as it is of the residents, and it is important to be sensitive to the difficulties that workers, as well as residents, face.

In the pages that follow, I offer an analysis of the dilemmas that confront nursing aides, exploring the roots of these dilemmas as well as their impact on aides and patients alike. I have tried to give a sense of what nursing home life looks and feels like for the nursing aides; at the same time, I have tried to guard against a romanticized view of the workers that ignores or passes over behavior that can harm patients. And though nursing aides are the central players, I also present the concerns of other groups in the nursing home, from patients and their relatives to higher-level nursing and administrative staff.

In trying to understand nursing home life, I am indebted, above all, to the staff of the New York City nursing home I studied. Although I cannot reveal the facility's identity, or the names of the staff, I owe a special thanks to many people there. The administrator went out of his way to help with my research, introducing me to staff, making information available, and offering acute observations of the structure of the facility. The director of nursing gave me assignments that placed me in strategic positions on the floors; many other professional staff, from social workers to the director of admissions, spent time helping me understand how the facility operated. Most of all, I want to thank the many nursing aides who tolerated my presence in the nursing home as I watched them work and asked endless questions and who were willing to give me time, during their meals and after work, to tell me about their jobs.

The research was made possible by a grant from the National Institute on Aging, 1 R15 AG08383-01. At the State University of New York, Purchase, Margaret Sullivan, now vice president for external affairs, made the grant application process relatively painless. A RISM Landes Senior Fellowship permitted me to take time off from teaching to finish the book. Thanks to Lambros Comitas, director of the Research Institute for the Study of Man, for his flexibility in the timing of the award. My thanks, as well, to Stanley Holwitz, at the University of California Press, for his enthusiastic support of the book.

Portions of chapter 7 have previously appeared in *Frontiers: A Journal of Women's Studies.* They are reprinted here with permission of the journal.

A number of friends and colleagues provided useful advice and criticism along the way. At the outset, Carroll Seron helped me to think through my ideas about the role of bureaucracy in the nursing home and commented on several draft chapters. I benefited from discussions with Susan Benson and other participants in the Women's Work Culture session at the 1991 American Anthropological Association meetings. Louise Lamphere read the entire manuscript and generously revealed her name as a reader for the University of California Press. Her comments, as well as those by the other, anonymous, reviewer, have helped in clarifying the arguments.

Once again, I owe a deep debt of gratitude to my mother, Anne Foner. Not many scholars have the good fortune to have a mother who is a leading figure in their field. My mother read many drafts of this manuscript with the kind of care and keen critical eye that I have become spoiled to expect. Given the long involvement of my father, Moe Foner, with New York City's major health care workers' union, it is perhaps fitting that I have come to write this book. Although he had no direct role in the research or writing of the book (indeed, the union representing workers in the nursing home I studied was not the one he is associated with), I like to think that some inspiration for the project came from my growing up in a household where issues of health care workers' union struggles were in the forefront.

Finally, thanks to my husband, Peter Swerdloff. He fielded endless queries about the project, from beginning to end, and helped me to crystallize many of the key ideas here. Alexis, my daughter, had to put up with an often distracted mother while I was writing the book and, toward the end, competition for use of the word processor as well. I dedicate this book to them.

1

Introduction

Millions of Americans have relatives in nursing homes, and those of us who reach an advanced age stand a good chance of living in one at some time. The people responsible for nearly all the direct patient care in nursing homes—helping frail elderly residents dress and eat and keeping them clean—are nursing aides. This book is about these workers: the contradictory pressures under which they work and the consequences for both workers and patients. On the one hand, there are high expectations that aides provide compassionate, supportive care. On the other, there are significant structural forces that often work against this kind of care.

The issue of nursing home care is of grave concern, especially as the percentage of the population in the oldest, most disabled age groups continues to rise and the number of nursing homes grows. According to a recent estimate, more than 40 percent of those Americans who turned sixty-five in 1990 will spend some time in a nursing home before they die (Kemper and Murtaugh 1991). Because the institutionalized elderly are so dependent on nursing aides, it is critical to know more about these paid caregivers—some 600,000 now working in the nation's nursing homes—who provide up to 90 percent of all the day-to-day care (Institute of Medicine 1986: 52; U.S. Department of Labor 1991).[1]

Largely ignored by the American public, when nursing aides do come to popular attention it is typically as uncaring and abusive actors in the "nursing home tragedy." Moreover, the bulk of the research on nursing home aides consists of brief statistical studies that give little feel for the workers' experiences, perspectives, and problems.[2] The handful of in-depth nursing home ethnographies look mainly at the dilemmas of patients, not workers.[3] In this book, aides are at the center, as I offer a view of institutional care through an analysis of the experiences and dilemmas of the paid caregivers who look after patients and who are, in truth, the backbone of nursing homes. Based on intensive fieldwork in a New York nursing home, this study gives voice to aides' concerns and expectations and reveals the complexities and difficulties involved in caring for weak and ill old people.

If the book illuminates important aspects of patient care, at the same time, it is more than a nursing home ethnography. The focus is on the nursing home as a work place, not just a residence. This is, in short, a study of work. Throughout, I am concerned with the special nature and demands of nursing home labor, and I draw and build on theories of work and bureaucracy as I try to understand and make sense of nursing aides' dilemmas.

Caregiving Dilemmas

What are the dilemmas nursing aides face in providing care for elderly patients? They are expected to see to patients' physical needs—what Jaber Gubrium (1975) calls "bed and body work"—and to do so with kindness and consideration. Detailed ethnographic study shows, however, that the nature of the nursing home environment makes it hard even for devoted workers to consistently offer sympathetic care.

Nursing aides are truly "in the middle," subject to contradictory pressures and demands from a variety of groups in the nursing home, each with its own interests and concerns: patients, administrators, nursing supervisors, patients' families, and co-workers. Aides face a number of caregiving dilemmas, as each of these constituencies poses a different set of problems and pressures.

In exploring the way these pressures impinge on nursing aides—and thus, indirectly, on patients as well—this study applies insights from the literature on industrial work and bureaucracy to the nursing home setting. In doing so, it calls attention to dimensions of nursing home life that have not been systematically explored and yet have crucial implications for patient care. Taking the lead from studies of industrial work, we can begin to see how important informal work cultures are for nursing aides and the many ways the home and family find their way onto the nursing home floor. At the same time, perspectives on bureaucracy suggest contradictions and tensions between the demands for bureaucratic organization and control, on the one hand, and the workers' desire for autonomy, on the other.

Of critical importance is that certain aspects of the nursing home bureaucracy and nursing aides' work culture can discourage sympathetic care. Some of the questions that arise are: How do bureaucratic demands of the institution affect the workers' ability to take the initiative in patient care and be responsive to residents' needs? What is the role of the aides' informal work culture in the nursing home setting? Does it make life more bearable for aides, and how does it affect patients?

The paradoxes and contradictions in the aides' work culture and the nursing home bureaucracy are especially dramatic, yet they should not obscure other significant dilemmas that plague aides as well. What emerges from my account is the enormous complexity of the difficulties aides confront, as they come from all sides, not just one or two sources. To appreciate the strains that aides must cope with at work, day by day, we must consider the full range of pressures they experience in their totality and the complex, and indirect ways these pressures affect nursing home patients. There is the structure of the nursing hierarchy, with aides uncomfortably on the bottom. There is the need to contend with patients' relatives, to say nothing of pressures from their own families. And, of course, there is the intricate mixture of attachments, obligations, and antagonisms involved in meeting the demands of frail and dependent residents. In all their relations at work, race, ethnicity, and gender play a role, providing important sources of solidarity among aides, yet also, at times, exacerbating divisions and tensions that arise with other groups in the nursing home.

Organization of the Book

I start out in chapter 2, by setting the stage and introducing the players. I present background material on nursing homes in the United States as well as on the particular facility I studied in New York City. An important issue is how typical this nursing home and the people who work there are of facilities and workers in the city and the nation as a whole.

The five chapters that follow focus, in turn, on the pressures aides confront from different constituencies in the nursing home and the way aides respond. I begin, in chapter 3, with the most obvious burden, patients. Caring for physically and mentally disabled residents entails enormous strains and difficulties and, often, literally, requires the patience of a saint. Chapter 4 explores the bureaucratic rules and administrative demands constraining nursing aides, the hidden injuries of bureaucracy, as I call them. Chapter 5 examines the impact of the direct agents of bureaucratic control, nursing supervisors. A key theme is the inequalities and strains in the nursing hierarchy, in which women (nurses) exercise authority over other women (aides). The pressures resulting from family relationships—both aides' own families and patients' families—are the subject of chapter 6. In chapter 7, I consider difficulties stemming from relations with co-workers. The emphasis is on the effects of the work culture that has developed among aides and the special dynamics and contradictions of work cultures in personal caring jobs.

The analysis of paid caregivers in nursing homes has broad implications for our understanding of long-term care, a topic that will be considered in the concluding chapter. Most critical: Are the pressures that discourage compassionate care an inevitable product of forces in the nursing home environment, or are they amenable to change? The conclusion also expands on theoretical questions that link the research to the literature on work. Theories of work in Western societies have largely been built on studies of industrial labor, a declining sector of the economy. There are relatively few studies of those who do "people work," the kinds of jobs that are becoming increasingly important in the economy. The analysis of nursing aides, who provide a particularly demanding form of "emotional labor," puts the dilemmas of service workers in sharp relief and sheds light on issues that have mainly been framed and elaborated with industrial employees in mind.

The Field Research

For eight months, in 1988–89, I immersed myself in the life of the Crescent Nursing Home, a 200-bed nonprofit skilled nursing facility in New York City. (The name of the facility, like all personal names used in this book, is a pseudonym.) I spent nearly all my time on the patient floors, in the world of the nursing aides.

This kind of in-depth fieldwork is, of course, the anthropologist's trademark. Of late, however, there has been much soul-searching in the discipline, what Clifford Geertz (1988: 71) calls "epistemological hypochondria" concerning "how one can know that anything one says about other forms of life is as a matter of fact so." The response to this question, as Sherry Ortner (1984: 143) suggests, is that we can only try to know "the other." "It is our capacity," she writes, "largely developed in fieldwork, to take the perspective of the folk on the shore, that allows us to learn anything at all—even in our own culture—beyond what we already know." My research at the Crescent Nursing Home offers a glimpse—filtered, inevitably, through the nature of my participation and interpretations—of the way nursing aides go about and experience their jobs and the problems that develop in this kind of paid caregiving.

Getting a start in the nursing home was not difficult, thanks to the cooperation of the administration. A week before I arrived, a letter, from me, was placed in every nursing aide's pay envelope explaining my role as an anthropologist who wanted to learn about their experiences. On my second day, the union delegate introduced me to the aides on each floor, assuring them that I was not working for the state or the administration and giving me a chance to answer questions about the project.

As a volunteer, I performed a wide range of chores that allowed me to observe and get to know aides on all the patient floors. To many residents, I was known as "the coffee lady" as I frequently served coffee in the morning to the dozen or so residents in the main dining room. Among my tasks on the floors where patients lived were wheeling patients to activities, making beds, helping patients eat at mealtimes, surveying personal items in patient rooms, straightening up supply closets, and organizing patient records. As the fieldwork progressed, I spent a lot of time simply watching aides as they did their jobs; a few allowed me to follow them around, pen and notebook in hand, recording what they did for the entire shift. Every day I spent breaks and mealtimes with nursing aides in their staff dining room. I attended special events like the annual Christmas party and went, with aides, to the regular in-service training sessions. With patients, I sat in on resident council meetings; with patients' relatives, family council sessions.

Observing aides over an extended period allowed me to see, at first hand, the way they interacted with patients (and patients' relatives), supervisors, and co-workers—how they carried out their work duties and coped with pressures from different groups in the nursing home. By being able to talk with and listen to aides, day after day, I heard their views and worries and learned how they reacted to concrete situations that arose on the job.

Initially, I gravitated to the Jamaican workers, especially at mealtimes. Given my previous research among Jamaicans, both in Jamaica and abroad, I felt comfortable with them, and they, too, were intrigued by someone who had spent time on the island (Foner 1973, 1978, 1987). It turned out that I knew the Jamaican politician-relative of one aide; and one of the dietitians had actually spent several months as a teacher-trainee in the village I had studied in Jamaica. After a month or so, however, I was equally at home having meals with groups of black American, Hispanic, and Haitian workers. Over the course of many months, I developed close ties with many aides of different ethnic backgrounds.

After a while, I became a kind of fixture of nursing home life. Aides got used to my being around and accepted, or at least generously tolerated, my presence. I was enormously flattered when toward the end of my fieldwork, one woman told me, "We all kind of take you for granted; it's like you work here now and are one of us." Of course, I was not one of them, and, as in any fieldwork situation, there were problems. Up until the very end, a few workers were suspicious of my motives, afraid, I think, that I would tell the administration what I heard and saw. Several had moments of ambivalence, as when one worker said, half in jest, that she would blow me up if I wrote in my book what I had just observed. And while I shared a bond with aides, as a mother and a woman, there was a racial, class, and cultural gulf that divided us. No matter how much time I spent with aides or how cordial or close our relations, I could not erase the fact that I was white, middle-class, professional, and American and that they were black and Hispanic, working-class, low-skilled, and, by and large, of immigrant background. My sojourn in the nursing home was temporary, too. Workers knew I would return to teaching, something they were not able to do.

In addition to participant observation, I carried out semistructured in-depth interviews with aides, outside the nursing home, to probe their occupational and personal backgrounds as well as their views on a wide variety of work-related topics. Some aides were eager to be interviewed and found time for me, after work, despite their busy schedules and long commutes. At the outset, I had hoped to interview about half the aides in the facility this way, but many were unable, or unwilling, to spare the extra time because of family responsibilities. In the end, fourteen agreed to be formally interviewed. Usually we went to a nearby coffee shop, and the interviews lasted about two hours. I was also able to informally interview another twenty aides in several sessions at meals and breaks and, occasionally, in brief periods on the job as well.

Although nursing aides were the focus of my interest, I did not restrict myself to interviewing them alone. I interviewed administrative staff and nurses on structural features of the nursing home as well as on their views of nursing aides. I became close to several alert patients who were willing to share their views of the facility and their caretakers with me. Not only did I listen to the woes and complaints of patients' relatives but, in a few cases, I was also able to talk to them, at length, outside the nursing home. And, finally, I mined various formal records to find out more about the way the nursing home worked and the situation of nursing aides, for example, nursing home records on admission statistics, the union contract, and nonconfidential records on employment tenure for nursing staff.

Given my close relations with so many nursing aides, it may seem strange that I often refer to them in this book by their last names, in a way that sounds formal, even distancing, to many Americans. It would not be odd at Crescent. Most aides, including close friends of many years standing, called each other by their last names. Usually, no title was used either. Louise Tait was "Tait" to all the nursing staff; Winnifred Hill, simply "Hill." "Ms." was added for a few older West Indian women, for example, Ms. McKenzie.[4] Out of respect, I always added Ms. when addressing workers who went by their surnames. This is the form I generally use in this study, although, of course, all names are fictitious to disguise the aides' identities. (Typically, patients were called by their last names as well, a pattern I also follow.) A number of aides, usually black American and Hispanic workers, were called by their first names, and I did this, too. In keeping with this practice, I use first names for some aides, only giving their full names when first introducing them.

Since I "officially" left the nursing home in 1989, I have been back many times to visit. Sadly, most of the patients I knew have died. A few of the aides I knew well are no longer there either, usually because they have retired. When I return and make my rounds of the floors to say hello to the workers, many invariably ask how my book is coming. Here, at last, in the pages that follow, is a full-length account of nursing home life from their perspective and with their dilemmas in mind.

2

Setting the Context: The Nursing Home World

American Nursing Homes: Trends and Changes

The nursing home industry has experienced phenomenal growth in recent decades, and it continues to grow as the demand for long-term care rises. Less than forty years ago, a 1954 Public Health Service inventory found a total of only 260,000 beds in 9,000 nursing homes in the nation which provided some degree of health services over and above room and board (Vladeck 1980: 43). By 1985, the numbers had soared to some 1.5 million beds in about 15,000 certified nursing homes.[1]

As nursing home beds have been added, so, too, have staff; by 1985, nursing and related care homes had the equivalent of almost 1.2 million full-time employees (Quinlan 1988: 7). Nursing homes now far outstrip general hospitals in numbers—there are two to three times more nursing homes than hospitals—as well as in patient beds and patient days (Johnson and Grant 1985: 3; Kane and Kane 1990). And public and private expenditures on nursing home care have soared. In 1989, nearly $48 billion was spent on nursing home care, close to four times the 1977 level (Short et al. 1992; Johnson and Grant 1985).

The virtual explosion of the nursing home industry is a result of several interconnected factors. Most prominent is that more and more Americans are living longer than ever before. Indeed, ours is an aging society, with a rapidly growing older population. Advances in medical care allow elderly patients to survive illnesses that once killed many. The increase in the number of those eighty-five years of age and older has been especially dramatic, more than tripling since 1960 to 3.3 million in 1990 (U.S. Senate Special Committee on Aging 1991). The "oldest old" are the very people most likely to be afflicted with chronic illnesses and physical ailments and in need of help with routine activities.

At the same time, demographic and social changes in the family system make it less likely that family members will be available to provide day-to-day care. Given increased geographic mobility, children are often scattered and inaccessible in times of need. Adult daughters, the traditional caregivers for the frail old, are increasingly likely to be working outside the home. And with the aging of the population, many children of the oldest old are themselves old and unable to physically manage their own and their parents' care at the same time. When care can no longer be provided at home, many elderly and their families turn to nursing homes because alternative forms of care in the community are unavailable or in short supply. Formerly, many old people with chronic psychiatric disorders went to public mental institutions, but since the deinstitutionalization of mental hospital patients and health policy changes in the 1960s, they now often end up in nursing homes (Johnson and Grant 1985: 80–82).

Public policy has played a key role in the nursing home expansion. Federal subsidies and loans for nursing home construction in the 1950s and 1960s, needless to say, stimulated the growth of nursing homes. And the enactment of Medicare and Medicaid programs in 1965 which provided health insurance for the elderly and indigent made it possible for a much larger proportion of the aged to use nursing homes. By the late 1980s, roughly 60 percent of nursing home residents had their care paid for by Medicaid.[2]

There is every indication that the nursing home industry will go on expanding, if at more modest rates than in the 1960s and early 1970s. Even if other long-term care services become more widely available, demographic trends make it certain that the demand for nursing home beds will continue to grow. Already, demand exceeds supply in most states; the number of nursing home beds is currently deliberately kept low by most states to control the growth of their Medicaid budgets (Institute of Medicine 1986: 5). (There was only a 10 percent increase in beds nationwide between 1978 and 1983.) In the next decades, the numbers needing long-term care will rise dramatically. According to conservative estimates, the population eighty-five years of age and older, more than one-fifth of whom now live in nursing homes, is expected to catapult from 3.3 million in 1990 to 4.6 million in 2000 and to more than 12 million in 2040 (U.S. Senate Special Committee on Aging 1991; Bould, Sanborn, and Reif 1989). One projection has it that the nursing home population will reach 2.1 million in 2005 and increase again to 2.6 million by 2020 (U.S. Senate Special Committee on Aging 1991).

The astounding growth in the population over age eighty-five is one factor involved in the changing character of nursing home patients: they are increasingly sick and disabled. Since modern nursing homes emerged in the 1960s, they have, of course, been filled with frail old people suffering from chronic physical illnesses, often combined with some degree of mental impairment. Today's patients, however, are likely to be older and sicker than those even a decade ago.[3] More, for example, are bedridden or wheelchair bound and need increasing amounts of personal and nursing care. In places like New York City, where the change has been especially dramatic, nursing home administrators talk of the redefinition of nursing homes as many facilities become more and more like "subacute" hospitals.

Clearly, there are pressures to admit a higher proportion of patients requiring extensive care due to the sheer enormity in the increase of the oldest old—pressures that will become more pronounced in the next few decades. Already, by 1985, the proportion of nursing home residents age eighty-five and older had risen to 40 percent, up from 35 percent in 1977 (Hing 1989).

Government health policy has also converged to create a sicker nursing home population. The prospective payment system under Medicare that was enacted in 1983 as a way to contain increases in hospital costs is key. Phased in over three years, this payment system reimburses hospitals a fixed amount per patient according to the Diagnostic Related Grouping (DRG) of the patient's condition. Hospitals have incentives to reduce lengths of stay and limit procedures to those for which expenses will be reimbursed. The result is that older hospital patients throughout the United States are being discharged "quicker and sicker" and are going to nursing homes in worse condition than before.

At the same time, Medicaid reimbursement policies adopted in a number of states have encouraged nursing homes to admit more seriously ill old people. Called case-mix systems for reimbursement, they give nursing homes financial incentives to accept heavy care patients by considering residents' illness level in reimbursement formulas.

Take New York, which introduced a case-mix reimbursement system in 1986. Before that time, nursing homes in the state were reimbursed under Medicaid on a per-patient basis, regardless of the level of care the patient required.[4] Given the nursing home shortage and clamor for beds, nursing homes could pick whom they would admit. They tended to prefer residents with low levels of need who required less service and were cheaper to care for. The new system, called the Resource Utilization Groups System, or RUGS, changed these preferences by rewarding nursing homes for taking in people with specialized medical needs. Now nursing home residents are classified in sixteen resource utilization groups, each representing a different category of care; facilities are reimbursed for direct patient care costs under Medicaid according to the average RUGS score of all patients. The larger the number of patients whose needs are judged most serious, the more money a nursing home is reimbursed under Medicaid.

Two years after the introduction of RUGS, the nursing home population in New York was noticeably sicker and more dependent; lighter care patients were being squeezed out, finding it harder and harder to get into a nursing home (Rudder 1989). One critic of the system speaks of a trend toward making nursing homes posthospital settings (ibid.). Reimbursement plans similar to New York's have been introduced elsewhere; by the end of 1992, fourteen states had some type of Medicaid case-mix reimbursement system.[5] According to a spokesman for a major nursing home association, "most states will eventually go this way" (Wolff 1987).

How Typical Is the Crescent Nursing Home?

These national trends are reflected in the institution where I did my research. The Crescent Nursing Home dates back to the early period of nursing home expansion in the 1950s. It has a rather tumultuous history, having begun as a profit-making enterprise, changing ownership several times, and, finally, in the 1970s, becoming a nonprofit facility. The nursing home is something of an anomaly in its gentrified neighborhood, located amid expensive apartment buildings and trendy boutiques and restaurants; many passersby who fail to notice the sign on the main avenue doubtless assume it is simply another old building recently converted into cooperative apartments.

Why did I pick this institution? As in most anthropological studies, it was a mixture of happenstance and forethought. Early on, in the planning stages, I had laid out some specific criteria. I was looking for a skilled nursing facility (with round-the-clock nursing care) of medium size where I could get to know most of the workers well and, at the same time, meet enough nursing aides to get a sense of their diversity.[6] I also wanted a "typical" New York City home where most patients were white and workers nonwhite. To simplify matters, the facility should have nursing units with similar numbers of patients and staff. Because of the early and late hours of the different shifts, I began my search with nursing homes that were fairly accessible to my home. Personal contacts led me to various nonprofit facilities. One that I was eager to study turned down my research request. One that was eager to have me turned out to be too unwieldy for the project: it had a wide array of special units and programs. When I approached the Crescent Nursing Home, it was clear that it fit my needs perfectly. The administrator was enthusiastic about the project and willing to go out of his way to help. I stopped my search and set the date for research to begin.

With regard to the question of how typical the Crescent Nursing Home is, there are two frames of reference: the nation as a whole and New York City. Crescent shares many features with nursing homes around the country, but it is also a product of its local environment. New York City, as the media constantly remind us, is special in many ways, and nursing homes there are quite different from the "average" U.S. facility in a number of respects.

Some basic nursing home characteristics make this clear. By nationwide standards, the Crescent Nursing Home is large (two hundred beds) and unusual in its ownership status (voluntary, not for profit). In 1985, three-fourths of the nation's nursing homes were profit-making enterprises, and only about one-third had as many as one hundred beds (Strahan 1987). In the New York City context, where nursing homes are larger and more frequently nonprofit, Crescent is less unusual. At the time of my research, two-thirds of the city's nursing homes had two hundred beds or more, and a little more than 40 percent were nonprofit (United Hospital Fund of New York 1988). Occupancy rates are high everywhere—99 percent at the Crescent Nursing Home and well over 90 percent in almost every state (Institute of Medicine 1986: 10).[7]

From a national or citywide perspective, Crescent is clearly an above average facility. Indeed, since substandard facilities are unlikely to welcome curious researchers, social scientists needing a nursing home's approval for intensive fieldwork projects are bound to study the better institutions. According to Crescent's administrator, the nursing home had been "in the dumps" when he arrived there in 1987 but, by 1989, was, overall, better than average. The medical, rehabilitation, and social work departments were definitely first-rate, while the administrator ranked the other departments, including nursing, as average. While the overuse of powerful psychoactive and antipsychotic drugs in American nursing homes is a modern-day scandal (Bishop 1989), the Crescent Nursing Home is scrupulous about avoiding unnecessary drugs to make patients more manageable. Less than one-fifth of the residents are given psychiatric drugs, and the number of medications per patient is very low as well, an average of four or less. The top administration is talented and well meaning, eager to create a model institution and sincerely devoted to trying to improve the quality of care.

As for Crescent patients, they fit the national profile in many ways: typically female, widowed, and white. Seventy percent of the facility's residents are women, about the same, it turns out, as the national figure.[8] Because women live longer than men, they run a greater risk of chronic disabling disease. And more women use nursing home care because more are widowed, a result of marital patterns in our society. Women tend to marry men who are older than they are, and, once widowed, women are much less likely than men to remarry.

Nationwide studies show that the risk of institutionalization is greater among old people without family support networks, the lack of a spouse being especially critical. Most Crescent residents, male and female alike, have no spouse, usually because of death but sometimes on account of divorce. Quite a few never married at all and have no children either. Several have outlived their children, while the surviving children of others often live far away. Sometimes a caretaking daughter is too ill herself to continue looking after her parent. And a great many residents are so infirm and incapacitated, with such complex medical needs, that caring for them at home involves enormous physical, emotional, and financial stresses that children (or surviving spouses) cannot handle.

Crescent patients are overwhelmingly—86 percent—white, with a sprinkling of Hispanics, blacks, and Chinese. This racial composition mirrors that of the local neighborhood, which has strong ties with and supplies most of the patients for the facility. The religious makeup of the nursing home also reflects the elderly population in the local area, heavily Catholic (about 50% of the residents) and Jewish (about 35%). The residents are very old—older, in fact, than the median age of eighty-one for the nation's nursing home population (Hing 1989). More than half of the facility's patients are over age eighty-five, and more than one-fourth are over age ninety. When I did my fieldwork, the oldest resident was 108; the youngest was a 51-year-old motorcycle accident victim, severely brain damaged and physically incapacitated.

That the Crescent Nursing Home is nonprofit and in an inner-city area, with a far from luxurious physical plant, probably explains why very few of the patients are paying with private funds (only 6% in contrast to one-third in the nation). The care of the rest is covered by government programs, with the vast majority receiving Medicaid and a few receiving Medicare.[9] Some entered as private payers but, after several years in the nursing home, spent down their assets and became eligible for Medicaid. Although now in severely reduced financial circumstances, most patients were formerly middle- or lower-middle-class citizens. They moved into the area when apartments were affordable for those with average means and when there were stable ethnic communities. Their occupations were diverse, ranging from beauticians and secretaries to musicians and teachers, and a few had been fairly prominent university professors and professionals.

The patient population at the Crescent Nursing Home is extremely ill and dependent. Although the most common ailments, diseases of the circulatory system and mental disorders, are those most prevalent in nursing homes throughout the United States, Crescent residents are more incapacitated, mainly due to New York's case-mix reimbursement system. There were very few patients with whom I could carry on a regular conversation, because most were too confused or too weak and ill. Hardly any could walk on their own or even with a walker; most could not eat without assistance; and nearly all were incontinent.[10] Nearly two-thirds had been diagnosed as having at least one mental disorder.[11]

The impact of the new reimbursement system on Crescent, as in most New York City nursing homes, has been dramatic. "It's like a restaurant getting a whole new clientele," is how the Crescent administrator put it. Now that hospitals are pressed by the DRG system, patients come to the nursing home from the hospital before they are fully recovered. The nursing home, itself under pressure to maintain adequate funding, selects patients who require substantial rehabilitation and nursing intervention to maintain a good RUGS score and reimbursement level.

New admissions need much more extensive attention than in the past.[12] More often, for example, they are bedridden and even semicomatose; more and more are tube-fed. No longer are the elderly with mental disorders like Alzheimer's disease admitted unless they have several physical problems. Because patients come in sicker, they stay a shorter time. The rate of rehospitalization is up, as some come in for a week or two, simply to return to the hospital. Many die soon afterward. The increasingly sick patient population has reverberations throughout the facility, from the dietary department, which must serve more pureed food and special diets, to social workers, who do more counseling with families rather than patients. The administration is concerned that nursing aides be increasingly skilled and observant now that they are dealing with the more seriously ill; nursing aides themselves have to minister to larger numbers of unresponsive patients with much greater care needs.

There are still a few relatively healthy, even some ambulatory, residents at the Crescent Nursing Home. A little more than 10 percent of the residents are protected under what is known as the "grandfather clause." Because they were admitted before RUGS went into effect, they can remain, even though by RUGS criteria, they should be transferred to facilities offering lower levels of care. As these residents slowly die, they will be replaced by more seriously ill old people so that the facility will truly be like a subacute hospital.

Like the patients they care for, nursing aides throughout the country are overwhelmingly female.[13] Indeed, when I was at Crescent, only two men worked as nursing aides, one a part-timer in the replacement pool who was dismissed soon after I left. This was out of a total of 95 aides: 75 with on-staff positions and another 20 "on call" in the replacement pool. Aides have low educational levels. The picture at the Crescent Nursing Home was much like the national view, where about one-third have completed less than twelve years of schooling (National Center for Health Statistics 1981).

Of profound importance is the marked racial divide between patients and aides at Crescent, a pattern that is becoming more common around the country as the number of minority aides continues to grow, especially in large cities.[14] *All* the Crescent nursing aides were black and Hispanic, hardly unusual in New York facilities given the city's enormous minority population. The only phenotypically white aide, a Puerto Rican woman, was viewed as Hispanic rather than white by most of her co-workers and administrative superiors.

Nursing aides reflect the special ethnic composition of their city's minority population. New York City is a major center of Caribbean immigrants in the country, and, not surprisingly, large numbers have gravitated to the nursing home field.[15] Black West Indians predominate among nursing aides at Crescent, as the figures on ethnic distribution on the day shift reveal (table 1). Of the fourteen nursing aides in the replacement pool who regularly worked during the day, five were black American, four Haitian, two Guyanese, two Puerto Rican, and one Ecuadorian. The night and evening shift aides were less ethnically diverse, with hardly any Hispanics and a much more dominant Jamaican presence.

Nursing aide turnover, a problem plaguing nursing homes nationally (where it is estimated to be 40 to 75% annually), is extremely low at Crescent and throughout New York City generally. In 1987 and 1988, the annual aide turnover rate at Crescent was as low as 5 percent.[16]

Aides stay put in New York City facilities because their wages and benefits are relatively good compared to those for other low-skilled jobs available to women in the city. Nursing aide jobs at unionized hospitals and nursing homes in New York City—the vast majority are unionized—are not easy to obtain. In fact, aides in the replacement pool at Crescent were willing to endure a two-year wait as part-timers to get on staff.

Clearly, this situation is not the case in most parts of the country where nursing homes are less likely to be unionized and wages and working conditions are much worse. A 1985 Bureau of Labor Statistics study of full-time nursing home aides in twenty-two metropolitan areas showed New York City ranking first in terms of average hourly wages (at $8.87). This far exceeded, by more than $2 an hour, the average wage in the second-ranking city, and it was over $5 an hour more than the worst-paid city (Quinlan 1988).

When I conducted my research, aides at the Crescent Nursing Home received $10.30 an hour for a 36 ¼-hour week, with an added

Table 1 *Ethnicity of Day Shift Nursing Aides*

	Number
English-speaking Caribbean	
Jamaican	13
Guyanese	3
Bermudan	1
Hispanic	
Dominican	6
Puerto Rican	1
Colombian	1
Black American	7
Haitian	3
N =	(35)*

* Includes all on-staff aides who worked on the day shift during my research.

10 percent for night and evening shift workers. In the same year in New York City, child care workers and attendants to the elderly in private homes averaged $5 to $6 an hour and garment workers about $7.50. "Not many places you will get $10 an hour, not bad for cleaning people's shit," is how one disaffected young Jamaican aide put it. Echoing most co-workers' sentiments, she added, "The money is the best thing about the job." Becoming a nursing aide was generally a step up from jobs Crescent workers had when they first came to New York. West Indians and American blacks from the South typically started out in New York in lower-paying jobs in private households—as attendants to the elderly, live-in baby-sitters, and domestics—where they were also isolated and subject to the whims of individual employers. Many Hispanic aides previously worked in New York factories in worse-paid and more insecure positions.

Benefits are another reason many came to the Crescent Nursing Home in the first place—and why they stay. Most important is major medical insurance coverage. Most opt for a health maintenance organization that covers virtually all their own, as well as uninsured children's and spouse's, medical costs. This is especially critical for the many women who support children on their own or whose spouses have no medical coverage. One particularly unhappy aide told me over and over how much she hated the job and wanted to leave. "The only reason I work," she said many times, "is for the health benefits."

There is an impetus to remain, too, to obtain benefits that hinge on seniority. Pension coverage vests after ten years, with retirement benefits increasing the longer one stays on the job.[17] Annual vacation leave is determined by length of service, beginning with one week during the first six months and going up, in increments, to five weeks after fifteen years. Vacation requests for particular times are also granted according to seniority. Holiday and sick leave benefits, though not linked to job tenure, are valued for the extra money they bring. Aides get fifteen days sick leave, with unused sick leave paid at the end of the year. When aides work on one of the twelve holidays—and all work on some—they receive a full day's pay plus time and a half, that is, two and a half times the regular day's wage.[18] If union-won wage increases and benefits motivate workers to stay on the job, the union contract also gives greater job security to those wishing to remain—and, much to the chagrin of management, makes it difficult to fire workers.

Given the low turnover rate, Crescent aides are older than the national average of thirty-four. Most are in their forties and fifties, and very few are younger than thirty. Large numbers are old-timers, around since the days when the nursing home was in private hands. One of the first nursing aides I met described herself as a "newcomer," having only worked at Crescent for sixteen years. Though many actually came after her, almost half of the on-staff aides had been at the Crescent Nursing Home more than fifteen years. Another fifth had been around for five to fifteen years, about a third between two and five years.[19] None of the on-staff aides had been at Crescent for less than two years (including time spent in the replacement pool). Since most were hired before New York State required specific nursing aide training, they simply learned what to do on the job. Newer recruits, hired in the mid–1980s, had taken short courses, lasting from two weeks to three months, to become certified;[20] after I left the nursing home, all had to (and did) pass a new clinical and written examination to meet new federal standards designed to ensure nursing aide competency.

National studies lament the many hardships caused by high turnover: aides leave with valuable knowledge of patients' habits and conditions; residents feel an emotional loss when staff members suddenly disappear; relations among remaining staff are disrupted when so many colleagues leave; and training, hiring, and supervising new aides exact a high financial cost. At the Crescent Nursing Home, management's concerns are exactly the reverse: they constantly complain about a "stagnating" work force that is resistant to change and, in some cases, too old for the physical demands of the job. "They've been here so long," said one administrator, "they've been running the units." Because aides have seen so many administrators come and go, there is a belief, as one high-level supervisor said, "that they'll be here tomorrow and I won't." The new administrators are determined to generate more turnover by building cases, through mandated disciplinary procedures, against aides who "do not make the grade." Numerous warnings were issued during my research, and three aides were forced to leave then or soon after. Ideally, administrators would like to hire aides who stay a few years en route to becoming licensed practical nurses (LPNs). Only two or three aides, however, were enrolled in LPN training programs;[21] the overwhelming majority were unlikely to leave voluntarily until retirement.

Structure and Organization at the Crescent Nursing Home

Like any institution, the Crescent Nursing Home has distinctive features that affect those who are part of it. The physical plant itself has a major impact on residents and workers. Whereas many facilities around the country were expressly built as nursing homes, Crescent inherited an aging and inappropriately designed physical plant. Numerous renovations have been made since the building was a women's residence—and since the facility was run for profit. When I was there, a new paint job and other decorative touches cheered up the place. The facility is clean, and framed posters brighten the halls and public areas. Still, offices, dining areas, and patient rooms are cramped, and there is a pressing need for more space. The building's landmark status, however, precludes certain alterations and additions, and there are financial limitations on what can be done.

The most serious problems are the extremely narrow halls and the lack of sufficient elevators. Traffic jams in the halls are not uncommon because only two wheelchairs can squeeze in width-wise at one time. Manipulating a wheelchair in the halls is difficult; walking can be treacherous for an unsteady resident, despite handrails. Two small elevators that can only fit two wheelchairs at a time service the eight floors (including the basement). (A service elevator connects the first floor and the basement; it can only be operated with a key and is mainly used for transporting supplies.) The sheer logistics of patient transport is an administrative nightmare. Patients must be ferried up and down the elevators to therapy, the main patient dining room, and various activities. For long periods at each mealtime, only one elevator is available since the other is used to bring food from the basement kitchen to the five patient floors. To make matters worse, one elevator is often out of service altogether, waiting to be repaired.

The seemingly endless elevator waits are a source of frustration for both patients and staff. It can take as long as twenty minutes for a wheelchair-bound patient to get a space in an elevator to go to therapy, over an hour to bring a group of patients downstairs to a special activity. Long lines of wheelchairs often clog the halls as patients wait for an elevator to get to lunch. Patients usually keep their complaints to themselves, but aides are more vocal, muttering about the time wasted hanging about for an elevator to get downstairs for breaks and meals—though, in truth, many could easily walk the few flights, and some use elevator waits as an excuse to extend time off from work duties.

One reason patients and staff spend so much time in elevators is that important services are on the main floor. There is the main patient dining room where the most competent, numbering about forty, eat lunch and dinner. A dozen or so also spend the morning hours there, watching television or just sitting, and several activities like religious services and special music performances are held in the main patient dining room as well. For nursing aides, the main floor is where they get their meals and take breaks, usually in the staff dining room. The only pay telephone in the building is on the main floor. So are staff locker rooms as well as most administrative offices, including the nursing department.

Patients also frequently go to the seventh floor: for therapy; for various activities like art classes; and to get their hair cut once a month. There is also a roof deck where residents can sit out in nice weather. Higher-level staff frequently "go to 7" because several administrative offices are there. The basement, the domain of the dietary department and some maintenance staff, is strictly out of bounds for patients, and nursing aides have no reason to go there.

The patients' and nursing aides' world is "on the floors." Most residents spend nearly all their time on the floor where they sleep; the most seriously ill rarely even leave their rooms. Each of the five resident floors has seventeen patient rooms for forty people. Most rooms have two to four patients; only three rooms on each floor are private. Since the doors to the rooms are almost always open, privacy is only possible when the curtains around each bed are pulled shut, something only a very few patients can do for themselves.

Furnishings in the patient rooms are sparse. Each resident has a bedside chest of drawers, a clothing locker, and a drawer by the common sink for toilet articles. There is also a chair for visitors. Above each bed is a bulletin board, often decorated with cards, pictures, and calendars, though those without regular visitors may have nothing there at all. About a third of the patients have their own television sets, often on all day at the aides' instigation. A few have radios, and a small number have their own telephones. Space shortages (as well as fear of theft) severely limit the personal belongings residents can keep, especially since two of the three small drawers available are reserved for the facility's towels and bedpans. Alert patients usually end up piling possessions on top of the chest of drawers, and some keep small quantities of food, brought by relatives, in the one glass bin the nursing home provides.

Each patient floor has a small dayroom where about a dozen residents eat lunch, several closet-size rooms for laundry, medical, and kitchen supplies, and four bathrooms (one reserved for staff). Whereas some nursing homes have staff lounges on the floors where aides work, there is no such space here which aides can truly call their own. Patients are generally in the dayroom, and the tiny nursing station is strictly the nurses' preserve. Some aides appropriate a particular patient's room as their "office," where they leave personal belongings like makeup and shoes and where they freshen up at the end of the day. While aides have a sense of propriety over their patients' rooms, ultimately these are the patients' spaces. When it is time to relax at breaks or mealtimes, aides hurry to leave the floor.

Beyond the basic physical environment, there is the actual structure of operations. For such a small institution, the Crescent Nursing Home is surprisingly complex, with more than a dozen departments and large numbers of staff, responsible around the clock for every phase of the residents' lives. There are actually more staff (222 budgeted positions) than patients, and 70 percent of the annual $12 million budget goes for salaries and wages.

Nursing is by far the largest department, with over 60 percent of the nursing home's staff, three-fourths of them nursing aides. The department is overwhelmingly female and minority; the director of nursing is herself a black Jamaican. Eight white American nurses—all registered nurses—spent some time in the nursing home when I was there;

by the time I left, only four remained, three of them part-time, including one agency nurse.[22] Apart from the two male nursing aides I mentioned earlier, only one other man worked in the department. He was a practical nurse, who resigned several months after I left the home.

The nurses are more of an ethnic mélange than the Caribbean-dominated aides. They come from Haiti, the Philippines, India, Jamaica, Costa Rica, Puerto Rico, Taiwan, and Nigeria, and there are several black and white Americans as well. Nurses also have a much higher turnover rate than aides: approximately 25 percent of the full-time staff nurses left in the year I did my research. Unlike aides, nurses at the time had a wide range of good jobs available to them given the nursing shortage in New York City.[23] A report in the late 1980s describes hospitals in a virtual bidding war for registered nurses (RNs), offering higher wages and more attractive conditions like flex-time (French 1989). Many nurses, the Crescent administrator told me, preferred to sign up with agencies for temporary positions, which offered high hourly wages (although no benefits) and the freedom to work when they wanted.

The director of nursing is definitely in charge of the department—formulating policy, hiring and overseeing staff, and preparing the budget, among other things. Below her is the gerontological nurse practitioner whose responsibilities include visiting hospital patients for preadmission screenings, following up on new admissions to see that nursing care plans are adhered to, and running the in-service education program. The other nursing administration positions changed in the middle of my fieldwork as part of a reorganization plan by the new director of nursing. Initially, there were two associate directors of nursing who evaluated, scheduled, and coordinated staff, but they were dismissed and replaced by new nurses, with new titles and assignments. A full-time administrative supervisor was now charged with keeping an eye on nursing staff on the five floors during the day; two part-time administrative nurses now worked in the nursing home four days a month, alternating as daytime weekend supervisors; and two other part-timers, on the job twenty-one hours a week, helped with staff coordination, auditing, and evening house supervision.

What the RNs, LPNs, and nursing aides do on the floors and how many patients they are responsible for depends a lot on which shift they work. When I arrived, the three shifts were 8:00 A.M. to 4:00 P.M. (day shift), 4:00 P.M. to midnight (evening shift), and midnight to

8:00 A.M. (night shift), but the times were pushed back an hour six months later to, respectively, 7:00 A.M. to 3:00 P.M., 3:00 P.M. to 11:00 P.M., and 11:00 P.M. to 7:00 A.M.

Nearly half the nursing aides and most of the RNs in the nursing home work on the day shift—working days, is how it is put. During this shift, the RN on each patient floor, the nursing care coordinator, has ultimate responsibility for the nursing staff and care of patients there. She schedules and evaluates staff and develops patient care plans that aides on all shifts must follow, deciding, for example, how to manage incontinence, treat bedsores, and use restraints. In the absence of a physician, she is the medical expert on the floor. As part of her routine, she handles certain medical procedures like inserting nastrogastric (NG) tubes. In fact, the nursing coordinator is swamped with state-mandated paperwork and spends most of her time sitting at the nursing station writing. For example, she must review medication records every day, update care plans, and record observations in nurses' progress notes.

With the exception of the sixth floor, there is also one LPN—officially called the charge nurse—on each floor during the day. The sixth floor has two LPNs because of its many seriously ill patients, a legacy from the previous nursing administration when it was the heavy care floor; now heavy care patients are assigned to all the floors. (Early on in my fieldwork, two RNs and one LPN worked on the sixth floor.) The charge nurse is busy much of the day giving and charting medications and changing dressings on bedsores and wounds. As she makes rounds to give medications, she also monitors more complex procedures like tube-feeding or the emergency use of oxygen. It is her job to check up on aides, schedule their daily work assignments, including morning and lunch breaks, and tell them to take and record various measurements, such as temperatures, when necessary. The charge nurse also supervises the serving of lunch on the floor. She has a substantial amount of paperwork, for instance, filling out part of the monthly summaries on each patient and nurses' progress notes.

Nursing aides on the day shift are involved in a full range of patient care. As Colleen Johnson and Leslie Grant (1985: 136) sum up, aides "lift patients out of bed, wash them, brush their teeth, bathe them, groom them, make their beds, change their soiled linen, clean up after them, dress them, escort them to the dining room, help feed them." Toileting patients involves taking them to the bathroom, offering a bedpan, or, most often, changing their incontinence briefs; when necessary, aides give enemas and collect specimens for the laboratory. Bedridden patients must be turned and positioned every two hours and the appropriate bedside chart filled out each time. Other regular paperwork includes recording bowel movements (daily) and vital signs (monthly); filling out an accountability sheet on a daily basis on the care given each patient; and completing an Intake/Output form (on fluids taken in and ejected) when, for example, a patient has a temperature or is on antibiotics.

When I came to the nursing home, there were four day shift nursing aides on every floor except the sixth floor, which had five. When the shift hours changed, all the floors were assigned five aides. (The additional aides came from other shifts and the replacement pool.) This staff increase reduced the aides' patient load from ten to eight, although they now had to serve breakfast, previously a night shift assignment. Unlike facilities in which aides regularly rotate among patients, at Crescent, when I was there, most on-staff aides had their own permanent sections (specific rooms and patients). To ensure seven-day staffing, there were also "floaters" on staff who rotated on one or two floors to cover for aides who had the day off. Even this did not meet staffing needs, and aides from the replacement pool were called to fill in for staff who were on vacation, off for the day, or called in sick. Hired in batches of about ten a year, twenty on-call aides made up the replacement pool. Since the day shift had the most on-staff aides—thirty-two in all when I left—more aides from the replacement pool were used during the day as well. There were especially large numbers of on-call aides on the weekends as on-staff aides were given alternate weekends off. In April 1989, for example, two to four on-call aides worked on the day shift on weekdays; ten to twelve were on duty on weekends.

Compared to other shifts, more demands are made on day shift aides, and even the administration agrees that they work harder. They serve two meals and have to rush to get patients ready for various morning activities such as therapy and religious services. "They have much more work and a much tighter schedule than the other shifts," one nursing coordinator explained.

And as one aide said, "There are more bosses around during the day." Day shift aides run the constant risk that administrators and other top-level staff will come onto the floor and walk into their rooms, sometimes specifically to check up on them. More senior nursing staff are around during the day; at least two nurses are always on each floor. Physicians make their visits during the day; administrators often wander in and out; therapists and other professionals are often on the floors checking records and patients; and state inspection teams come at this time. Because they have so much to do and because they work under the eyes of the administration and so many superiors, day shift aides have less time to sit and chat with each other on the job. Certainly, they cannot, like night shift aides, even think of nodding off for a few minutes' sleep during work hours.

Despite these drawbacks, most day shift workers prefer their hours. As one aide told me, "I want to be beneath my sheets at night." They worry about the safety of traveling at night; and some prefer to work when patients are awake and can talk to them. Aides with young children like to be at home to care for them in the late afternoon and evening. My own child care arrangements meant that I spent most of my time on the day shift, so the day shift aides—their routines, interpersonal relations, perspectives, and life stories—were those whom I came to know best.

On the night and evening shifts, there are far fewer nurses in the facility. One LPN is in charge of each floor. She gives out and charts medications, checks and makes notes on patients, and supervises the nursing aides. The RNs in the facility—one on the evening shift and one on the night shift—are house supervisors, based in the nursing office, who make rounds of the floors as they coordinate and monitor nursing care, confer with charge nurses, and are on hand if emergencies arise.

The night shift consists of a skeletal staff, with an average of two aides per floor (and eighteen aides altogether on staff). Each aide is responsible for twenty patients; residents are asleep most of the time, and compared to the daytime, they require relatively little care. This is the only shift that gives no baths, serves no meals, and does not routinely dress or undress patients. Aides make regular rounds to check on patients, which sometimes involves changing or turning them, and there are frequent calls from patients with various requests. When the night shift aides left work at 8:00 A.M., breakfast was their responsibility—an enormous burden, they felt, as they had to rush to feed twenty patients each when they were tired and eager to end their shift. When the hours changed to 11:00 P.M. to 7:00 A.M., however, they were relieved of this job, which was turned over to the day shift aides, who grumbled about the extra burden of serving two meals.

Evening shift aides arrive in the late afternoon, in time to give some baths, feed patients dinner, and change and toilet residents and get them to bed. Their patient load runs from ten to fourteen. Typically, there are three or four aides per floor on weekdays and three on weekends, with a total of twenty-four aides on the evening staff. They are especially busy in the first five or six hours on the job, but toward the end of the shift, when many residents are asleep, the floors are relatively quiet. In general, after 5:00 P.M., when administrative, professional, and office staff have gone home, the pace of the nursing home is slower and the atmosphere, for the workers at least, more relaxed.

Like day shift aides, night and evening workers have become accustomed to and generally prefer their hours. Many have other commitments during the day, such as additional jobs or school. They certainly appreciate the extra 10 percent wage differential they get for working irregular hours. And as one woman said, "I don't have the administration on my back." "At night," she continued, "nobody is after you. In the day, you have to get the patient ready to go right away to OT [occupational therapy] or downstairs to lunch. At night you work your own way; take it slow, take it fast, do it your own way."

The two other big departments in the nursing home, housekeeping and food services, are filled with service workers. Nursing homes are bottom heavy, with enormous numbers of low-skilled workers and a small percentage of professionals. At Crescent, nursing aides alone make up more than two-fifths of the entire staff, and housekeeping and food service workers—who clean the nursing home, organize supplies, and cook the food—comprise another one-fifth.

Service workers throughout the facility (including nursing aides) have much in common. In addition to filling the lowest prestige and lowest paid jobs, with roughly similar wages, service workers are almost all people of color. They wear uniforms on the job, a symbol of the dirty work they do, in contrast to higher-level staff who work in street clothes (with a white coat over them, in the case of the medical director and registered nurses). Service workers eat and take breaks in the staff dining room; few higher-level staff, who have offices to retreat to, ever stay there.

Network hiring has led to particular ethnic configurations in the different service work departments. Housekeeping employees—cleaners and maintenance and supplies workers—are nearly all Hispanic, primarily from the Dominican Republic. While nursing aides are predominantly English-speaking West Indians, food service workers are a mix of Dominicans, Jamaicans, and black Americans.

If the nursing aide job is a female bastion, other service work is a male domain. All but three housekeeping employees and one kitchen worker, who serves staff meals, is male. (The nursing home contracts out laundry services so that the women responsible for laundry and linens handle distribution in the facility.) One porter is assigned to clean each patient floor, adding a regular male (and Dominican) presence to the floor work force. While nursing aides work around the clock on three shifts, almost all other service workers are concentrated in the daytime. Focused on meal preparation, the kitchen is active from early morning to early evening, and nearly the entire housekeeping staff works during the day.

At the top of the occupational ladder, the administrators and department heads, who run the nursing home and make important decisions, are distinguished by race: almost all are white.[24] Interestingly, the few exceptions include the heads of housekeeping, nursing, and food services, who supervise departments with enormous numbers of minority service workers. In general, most professionals outside of nursing are white, adding to their social distance from service employees.

Because of the nature of their jobs, quite a few of the professional and administrative staff—for example, the accountant, the maintenance director, and the head of admissions—have almost no contact with patients or nursing aides. The administrator, who is responsible for the overall management of the facility, and his two assistants are generally closeted in their offices or at meetings. Professionals who work with patients inevitably come into contact with aides, but their attention is focused on patients' problems, and they tend to have an off-hand manner with aides. Often, they ignore aides altogether as they go about their jobs; sometimes they give aides a brief nod of recognition or greeting. Rarely do conversations arise, and when they do, they are usually strictly about business.

"Our role is to be patient advocates," is how one of the three social workers described his position. Social workers walk a fine line, trying to help patients and their families who come to them with problems but also aware that success hinges on not antagonizing the nursing staff. The social workers do, in fact, tend to maintain amicable, though distant, relations with nursing aides. Often, they help with difficult patients. Social workers are called in by nurses, often at the aides' request, when, for example, patients refuse to be washed, will not have their rooms cleaned, or are physically violent. When a complaint is voiced by patients or their families, social workers are careful to indicate their understanding of the aides' problems and sensitivities—and to take them into account—as they try to work out a solution.

The three physical and occupational therapists and their four assistants are nearly always on the seventh floor, where the twenty-five rehabilitation patients go for therapy. Occasionally the therapists come to the patient floors to check records and make rounds, but they have little to do with aides. The director of volunteers, who runs an active program, rarely comes to the floors and spends her time recruiting and scheduling volunteers who help out in the home. Nor do aides have much contact with those who run patient activities—the activities director and her assistants, volunteers like art teachers, and the part-time pastor. Most activities take place off the patient floors and, in any case, involve only a small minority of residents. A part-time music therapist visits each floor once a week to run a group sing; to many aides, this is simply another burden, requiring them to wheel patients to the dayroom for the activity. A kind of wandering troubadour, guitar in hand, the music therapist also regularly comes to serenade room-bound residents with their favorite songs, which patients and even many aides seem to enjoy.

Physicians are familiar figures on the patient floors. The Crescent Nursing Home has what is known as a closed services medical system, instituted a few months before I arrived. On admission, residents are assigned one of the five on-staff physicians, who is affiliated with a nearby voluntary hospital. He supervises their care in the nursing home and if they are hospitalized. Each physician is responsible for forty patients on one floor and works in the home 17½ hours a week. Every day the "floor physician" sees patients he has been asked to look at; staff members note in the problem list any condition they want the physician to check. In any case, the doctor examines every patient at least once a month and orders medications as well. The doctors' relations with the aides are formal and distant, and whatever criticisms they have they keep to themselves. In addition to coming every weekday for a few hours, the physicians rotate weekend and on-call assignments among themselves and with the full-time medical director.

Also, consultants—a podiatrist, an ophthalmologist, a psychiatrist, an ear-nose-and-throat doctor, a surgeon, and a dentist—regularly visit the nursing home to examine patients.

Finally, as part of their job of planning patients' meals, the two dietitians come to the floors to look at medical records and weights, check patients' food preferences, and observe mealtimes. The white dietitian, having little in common with and somewhat contemptuous of the aides, only speaks to them when specific food questions arise. The Jamaican dietitian, however, often stops to chat and gossip with Jamaican aides, some of whom she knows from her days back on the island. Indeed, it turned out that we had mutual acquaintances in Jamaica, since she spent time as a teacher trainee in the village I studied. These contrasting relations of the dietitians with the aides illustrate how important race and ethnicity are in staff interactions and foreshadow themes that will come up in later chapters.

3

Patients: Pressures, Frustrations, and Satisfactions

Caring for nursing home patients is difficult, demanding, and frustrating. Many are suffering from severe dementia; most are confused to some degree. Their physical ailments are severe, and they do not get better. Some are completely unresponsive, while others are bitter and hostile. In short, residents' physical and mental condition and their need for enormous attention and assistance are a never-ending source of pressure for nursing aides.

How do nursing aides cope with and respond to patients' demands and their physical and mental ills? The nursing home literature generally offers a bleak view. It is filled with horror stories about staff who neglect and abuse patients. Even many ethnographic reports recount gruesome details. Jeanie Kayser-Jones (1990), for instance, characterizes employees at the California nursing home she studied as frequently "authoritarian and indifferent in their dealings with patients" and as showing "little concern for their dignity and individual rights." Staff infantilized, depersonalized, dehumanized, and victimized residents. Other studies depict aides as condescending, curt, and cruel, often treating residents like inanimate objects and insensitive to their needs (Fontana 1977; Gubrium 1975; Vesperi 1983). The Tellis-Nayaks (1989) speak of personal care without commitment: soulless service with a cheerless attitude and cold touch.

This overwhelmingly negative impression is misleading. Admittedly, abuse, insensitivity, and meanness were all too common at the Crescent Nursing Home. But this is only part of the story. Less frequently mentioned in the literature is that aides themselves are victims of abuse from patients. And instead of focusing only on abuse and mistreatment, we also need to look at the positive aspects of patient care. Despite the relentless emotional and physical demands patients make on Crescent aides, many are truly kind and caring to residents and conscientious in their work.

Patients' Condition and the Daily Routine

The basic tasks in a typical day shift schedule sound, on the face of it, straightforward and simple. One aide summed it up: "In the morning, I get patients up and dressed and make beds and give one or two baths or showers. Then lunch. I feed people in the dayroom and bring trays to those eating in their rooms and help them. After my lunch, I change patients and put back to bed those who want to go and then do my paperwork."

This brief summary glosses over how physically straining, emotionally wearing, and dirty the work is—and how patients present problems every step of the way. What seem like simple operations, such as changing a patient's undergarments, often involve considerable physical effort and special techniques to coax and cajole residents to cooperate. And "other little knickknacks," as one worker called them, come up during the day. A patient may ask to be moved, for example, or regular duties such as taking monthly weights or temperatures must be carried out.

Each task presents its own difficulties. Getting patients up in the morning requires continual bending, lifting, and pushing. Only a few residents can wash and dress themselves; most need total, or near-total, assistance. The routine goes like this: an aide washes a patient's body (while scanning for bruises or other physical changes), applies Vaseline or lotion to sensitive parts, and puts new incontinence briefs on. She dresses the resident and puts her in a wheelchair, often with a mechanical lift. She then finishes the remaining toiletries such as brushing hair and checking (and if necessary, cutting) nails. Every morning, an aide gives one or two baths, a procedure that takes 35 to 45 minutes per patient.

Lifting is the worst physical strain. Even with mechanical aids, it is very taxing. The type of mechanical lift used at the Crescent Nursing Home requires continual cranking, and it does not eliminate the need to lift patients manually to position them correctly in their wheelchair. Since there is only one lift per floor, its use is reserved for patients who are the most difficult to get in and out of bed. Patients who can offer help in standing up and being moved do not require a mechanical lift. Usually, however, they require some manual lifting. This is strenuous even when residents are thin, and aides commonly complain about back pain. Lifting patients by hand, in and out of wheelchairs, is a delicate operation, for the slightest bumps can bruise elderly residents' fragile skin.

Worst of all are immobile patients who are "stiff like brick" and offer absolutely no help. Lifts are used for these patients, but getting them in the right position to put into a lift is difficult, as is turning them from side to side in bed for washing and dressing. "I can't lift that man," complained a Jamaican aide, referring to a heavy "deadweight." "I come in here with all my organs, and I want to leave with all of them." Changing him was an ordeal, and he constantly slipped down in his chair, requiring manual lifting to be repositioned. One extremely contracted ninety-one-year-old woman, who entered the home malnourished and suffering from severe dementia, stayed in bed all day, curled up in a fetal position. Just washing her and changing her linens was a problem. The aide had to position her numerous times, slightly raising her to pull the old sheet out from under and lifting her again to put a clean sheet on. All the while, the resident wailed, emitting truly horrible moans and cries.

Bowel work, as Gubrium (1975: 139) calls it, is part of nursing aides' routine. They are used to cleaning residents' stools. Talk about the kinds of bowel movements patients have had, or their state of constipation, is common. Yet as Gubrium notes of Murray Manor, "When bowel work is particularly disgusting, floor personnel are disgusted." No aide relishes having to cope with the smell, mess, and continual cleaning and changing required by severe diarrhea. Aides also find it repugnant and more work when residents play with their feces. Selma David, an eighty-two-year-old woman with severe dementia, was known for doing this. After being washed and dressed, she often smeared feces all over her body, requiring a shower and, obviously, new undergarments and clothes.

Apart from the physical strains and difficulties, patients may rant or scream while aides try to wash and clothe them. Some actively resist. And some, usually through no fault of their own, undo work aides have already done. Patients suffering from dementia may try to pull off their clothes. The confused and incontinent frequently soil or wet themselves soon after they are cleaned.

One afternoon, Nina Acosta, a kind and considerate young Dominican aide, was completing her tasks for the day by changing Ms. David in the bathroom. Nina stood Ms. David by the sink, holding onto her for support while trying to wash her bottom with soap and water and put on new incontinence briefs. This was no easy task. Ms. David babbled incoherently and writhed all the while. No sooner did Nina finish, with relief, than Ms. David cried out, "I have to go, I have to go, it's running down, it's running down." Nina had to start the whole procedure from scratch.

Residents are often frightened of having their nails cut, and the very confused can get into a state when an aide pulls out her scissors to begin the job. Constant comforting and reassurance usually does the trick, but when patients continue to wriggle and yell, the job is more difficult and time-consuming. "Don't do it to me, don't do it to me," one resident screamed as she flailed her arms about. Another aide helped by holding down the resident's arms, but, even then, cutting her nails took nearly fifteen minutes to complete.

Helping residents eat is a wearing process when they must be fed spoonful by spoonful and they are slow or resistant. When I left the nursing home, much of the day shift's time was taken up with serving food: breakfast, lunch, and food supplements to some residents in the afternoon. Feeding frail sick people, as Timothy Diamond (1988: 45) observes, involves delicate tasks that require much skill—learning their pace, knowing how to vary portions and tastes, and figuring out how to communicate nonverbally while feeding. Aides are under pressure to complete meal assignments within strict time limits; they also know that nurses and dietitians monitor residents for weight loss and dietary intake. Residents who are confused, angry, depressed, or simply loath to eat the unappetizing food can make mealtimes an ordeal.

Some residents, out of confusion or willfulness, refuse to eat at all. Physical disabilities make it hard for some to swallow and cause others to spit or cough up their food. In the dayroom, I saw many demented residents throw food or reach into a neighbor's tray to grab handfuls of servings. Screaming, yelling, and whining are common. Ida Rubin had deteriorated badly during my stay. She suffered from advanced Alzheimer's disease and weighed less than seventy-five pounds. When I, or an aide, fed her, she whined and cried and continually pushed us away. It was difficult to coax her to swallow more than a few bites.

I found slow residents especially trying. On many Tuesdays, I fed Ms. Cantor, a woman in her nineties with a severe form of dementia. When she used to have lunch in the dayroom, she ate poorly; with a full-time volunteer in her room she did much better. She was, however, excruciatingly slow, taking over an hour to eat lunch. I sat with her, pouring her drinks, cutting her food, and handing her spoonfuls, but each bite seemed to take forever for her to chew. Occasionally she muttered a few incomprehensible words, but mostly she stared at me, every once in a while smiling or bursting into laughter.

Throughout the day, residents, understandably, make constant demands. Helpless in their beds and wheelchairs and frustrated by their dependence, the physically weak but more mentally alert are especially likely to want things: to be changed or moved, for example, or have a glass of water or assistance in reaching a magazine or newspaper. "He's much too alert," was a Jamaican aide's comment about Mr. Wood, who continually summoned aides to change or reposition him or to make sure his medications were given on time. Day shift aides have eight to ten patients to look after. "When one want you to be there all the time, how you gonna do it?" Residents, of course, have a different perspective. "You can't understand what it's like," said Ms. Calhoun in one of her lucid periods. "I have trouble wheeling myself, and sometimes I start to cry when I'm left in the middle of a room." Pleas to go to the bathroom ring through the halls—"I don't know if I'm going to make it, nurse, nurse"—as confused residents have real, or imagined, fears of wetting or soiling their undergarments.

Many residents simply crave attention, like Helen Nichols, a former commercial artist, now suffering from acute dementia. She tried to buttonhole anyone who passed in the hall. "Come here for a minute, sweetheart," she would say. "I want to talk to you. I just have one thing to tell you."

Demented residents frequently cry, plead, and moan. Ms. Nichols often demanded to go to the subway; another woman on her floor cried in the halls about her baby, "Don't leave me, don't leave me." On the second floor, a woman regularly positioned herself by the nursing station where she intoned, "When are we going outside, when are we going outside?" for what seemed like hours on end.

Those with extremely short-term memories commonly ask the same question over and over, even after they have been answered. Evelyn Frank could not remember that cookies were no longer served with morning coffee in the main dining room. When I arrived with the coffee, she inevitably asked for a cookie. Every day, I went through the same explanation. And every day, no sooner did I explain than she asked again and again.

If aides are assaulted by constant pleas for help, some residents are disconcerting for exactly the opposite reason: they are comatose or semicomatose and completely (or almost completely) unresponsive. No matter what the aide does, they never react. "Just like there, not even a yell or scream," explained one worker. "You can't even know if you hurt them or they're in pain."

However good their care, the fact is that with very few exceptions, residents inevitably deteriorate and eventually die. (A very small number leave the facility to return to their own homes or to enter institutions that offer "lower levels of care.") Many aides quietly grieve when residents they were close to die. A couple now defended themselves against becoming too emotionally involved after experiencing deep sorrow at the death of a favorite. "There was one patient who was here, I was very close to her," Elaine Rogers told me. "She used to call me her daughter, and she died. And from that. . . . One reason you can't get too emotional, when they die you feel it too much. When Betty die I feel it so and I say never again, never again."

Worker Abuse

To add to aides' problems, there is abuse from residents, ranging from angry comments to physical violence. "Curse you, scratch you, bite you," one aide summed up. A few residents, as Mila Aroskar and her colleagues (1990: 282) note, are manipulative by nature. Others take out their anger and unhappiness on aides or dehumanize workers to regain control over their living environment. Most abusive residents suffer from mental impairments and are not responsible for their actions.

Crescent aides are aware that most abusive residents "do not know what they are doing"; they reserve their heartiest dislike for residents who "have their senses and are nasty." Still, conscious or not, the effect is the same. Aides have to deal with the resulting scratches, punches, yells, and insults. And they do not like it (see Savishinsky 1991: 164, 169, on this "hidden side of nursing home life" in the facility he studied). To many aides, abusive patients are the most difficult ones. "I understand it, but I don't like when the patient abuse me," as one aide put it. "I been scratched a few times. What can I do? They don't know what they doing. Not because they don't like you."

Every aide has stories to tell about the battle scars received during the course of duty. Sitting at lunch one day, a group of Jamaican aides joked about how one patient knocked some teeth out of Ms. Wright's mouth and how another bit Jocelyn Edwards on the arm and hand. Despite help from two aides, Ms. Rios, a Dominican aide, was badly scratched one morning—she sustained a bleeding and swollen patch on her arm—by a resident who thrashed and scratched in the bath. The nurse finally requested that the doctor order a sedative for this resident to calm her down before her weekly bath.

Sexual overtures and fondling from residents are common. Aides tend to laugh off such actions from confused residents, but they are often hostile if the resident is alert. "I can't stand that man," said one aide, referring to a patient deemed to be "90 percent all there." "He put his hands all over you. Now Welch, he massages your thighs when you wash him, but he don't know what he's doing." Another aide said she was initially horrified when after washing a resident known to be a lesbian, the woman loudly proclaimed, "You fucked me, now you want me to fuck you?" "I ran to tell the nurse," the aide explained. "I said I have something to tell you. And she said, 'Oh yeah, she does that all the time.'"

Then there are the insults, name-calling, swearing, and even threats of blackmail. Many times, I heard residents shouting and screaming at their aides. "You fucking bitch, you fucking bitch," one woman yelled venomously the entire time she was being dressed. Perhaps the most difficult resident in the nursing home was an immensely fat sixty-five-year-old schizophrenic, who sat naked in her bed all day. She covered every surface of her bed, drawers, and floors with used cups, utensils, napkins, and food—refusing to have them cleaned—and yelled in deep stentorian tones whenever an aide came near and tried to wash her. In my role as a volunteer, I was also a target for abuse from residents. On several occasions, I was assigned to Mr. Hammond at lunchtime. He was able to eat by himself but needed considerable help. Frustrated when he dropped food or could not manage his sandwich, he took out his anger on me, screaming and cursing in a loud barking voice, "Damn you, damn you, can't you get anything right?" Another resident, Harriet Brandt, was an alert woman who kept an eye on my morning coffee-giving activities in the main dining room.

Once, when someone asked me for a second cup and I was about to oblige, Harriet angrily threatened to report me if I acceded to the request.

Patients can lash out with racial slurs as well, something aides are too sensitive about to laugh off. Aides feel that even demented residents who "curse you black" must have harbored racist sentiments in their healthier years if they use such epithets now. Workers told me many stories of residents calling them "nigger bitch" or "monkeys." "You say good morning to Mr. Buckley," a Jamaican aide said, "and he say, 'Go away from me you black nigger.'" On a number of occasions I heard this kind of abuse, as when one resident screamed out at her black Jamaican aide, "The whites are all right but not the blacks."

Aides' Response: Saints or Monsters?

Clearly, having to cope with this kind of abuse and the physical and emotional strains I have described can try anyone's patience. Unlike adult children who look after frail elderly parents, nursing aides are not bound to residents by long years of love and affection. Nor, as is often the case with caregiving children, do they feel they owe the elderly a debt for services rendered in earlier years. Aides are paid to do the job of caring for strangers. And racial and ethnic cleavages create additional barriers and misunderstandings between aides and residents.

While continual contact with the same residents day after day fosters closeness, it can also magnify tensions. Residents' habits and idiosyncrasies can become extremely grating. Even though the aide may dislike the resident passionately, the aide must dress, bathe, massage, and feed her or him.

One response to patients' demands and abuse is the kind of insensitive and cruel treatment so often chronicled in the nursing home literature. Another response is understanding and compassionate care. In fact, most Crescent aides fall somewhere in between: they are neither saints nor monsters.[1] Only a very small minority are consistently cruel or consistently warm and supportive. Most aides are generally kind and helpful to residents, although at times they lose their tempers and behave in ways that come across as mean. And many establish relations with residents that they and the patients find gratifying.

ABUSE AND ILL-TREATMENT

First, consider the negative side of the aides' response to patients. Abuse, we know, is distressingly common in American nursing homes. Karl Pillemer and David Moore's (1989) quantitative study reveals alarming figures.[2] Of the 577 nursing home aides and nurses they interviewed, 36 percent said they had seen at least one incident of physical abuse in the last year; as many as 10 percent reported that they themselves had committed one or more physically abusive acts. Most common was the use of excessive restraints or pushing, grabbing, shoving, or pinching a patient. Psychological abuse was even more widespread. Eighty-one percent said they had seen at least one incident in the preceding year such as yelling, insulting, or swearing at a patient. Forty percent admitted to having been psychologically abusive on at least one occasion.

Although I did not systematically count instances of abuse by nursing aides at the Crescent Nursing Home, physical abuse—acts carried out with the intention or perceived intention of causing physical pain or injury to another person (Straus, cited in Pillemer and Moore 1989)—was rare. The most frequent type of physical abuse reported in Pillemer and Moore's study, excessive use of restraints, was largely out of the nursing aides' purview: nurses, not aides, ordered restraints. While I occasionally heard about or observed cases of pushing, grabbing, pinching, or shoving, aides were careful not to physically harm residents because this could get them in serious trouble and, ultimately, cost them their jobs.

Aides tended to vent their anger and irritation at patients through psychological abuse—acts carried out with the intention or perceived intention of causing emotional pain to another person (ibid.). Psychological abuse was informally tolerated on the floors at the Crescent Nursing Home, and as a result, it was common. Even so, only a handful of aides were consistently abusive in this way. Statistical as well as qualitative studies of neglect and mistreatment do not stress that the very same workers who are abusive one moment may be considerate and kind the next. Of the thirty-five on-staff nursing aides I closely observed on the day shift over many months, only four were abusive and mean more often than not. Another four were often indifferent, sullen, and unresponsive. Of the rest, four, as far as I could tell, never intentionally mistreated patients. The remaining twenty-three were occasionally psychologically abusive or unkind. The word "occasionally" must be emphasized. Most of the time, these aides stifled their irritations and, despite provocations and pressures from patients, were sympathetic and caring.[3]

As in Pillemer and Moore's study, yelling and swearing at and insulting patients were the most frequent forms of psychological abuse at Crescent. Ms. Riley was guilty of all three, in my view one of the four worst day shift aides. A big, heavy-set Jamaican woman in her early fifties, she had been at Crescent for about six years, having previously worked, on and off, as a nursing aide for a private agency. Among her Jamaican co-workers, Ms. Riley was a definite presence. She held forth at lunch, telling hilarious stories and responding to comments with quick and clever humor. I, too, loved to hear her talk, and she was especially friendly to me because of our shared Jamaican connections. To patients, however, she was terrifying. If looks could kill, hers would, and she often yelled in loud, cruel, and angry tones. "You better shut up or I'll fix your ass. Eat your food," she screamed at a whining patient in the dayroom who was slow to eat. When a resident, in her own room, asked for a cup to spit into, Ms. Riley barked, "Is your spit, housekeeping will come to clean it up." As she left the room, Ms. Riley glared at the resident and said, with vehemence, "You bastard." To another complaining resident, Ms. Riley yelled, "I don't have to listen to you or look at you."

Often, yelling at residents occurs after a concerted but ultimately ineffective effort to keep one's temper under control. Rosa Sanchez, an older Dominican aide, was generally considerate and concerned with the patients' welfare. One of her residents, Ms. Kelly, was extremely difficult. She constantly screamed and yelled, coughed and spit up phlegm, and roughly grabbed passing nurses and aides. One afternoon, Rosa was taking pains to coax Ms. Kelly to eat and calm down. Each time Rosa tried to get her to take a bite, Ms. Kelly flailed and loudly shrieked. This, in turn, induced terrible coughing fits and spitting. After about ten minutes, Rosa reached the breaking point. She put her hands to her head and yelled, "Shut up, shut up you. Oh my pressure [Rosa has hypertension], this is giving me pressure."

The other indicators of psychological abuse that Pillemer and Moore used in their study—isolating a patient beyond what was needed to control him or her, denying a patient food or other privileges as part of a punishment, and threatening to hit or throw something at a patient—were rare at the Crescent Nursing Home. Unfortunately, other forms of mistreatment were not. One of these was taunting and teasing patients and making jokes, in front of them, at their expense. When Ms. Riley asked Mr. Adams, "Where's Valerie?" one afternoon, this was deliberately cruel. Ms. Riley found it amusing that Mr. Adams, in his confused state, began to look expectantly for his wife, Valerie, even though Ms. Riley knew full well that Valerie would not be coming that day. Later on, she nastily joked to him, "You're terrible, right?" Sometimes groups of aides ganged up to tease a resident. One morning three aides were in the elevator with Mr. Langdon, an alert wheelchair-bound resident. They loudly laughed among themselves about how badly he smelled. "He needs a fire hose to clean him down," one commented.

Then there are the cold stares and withering looks aides direct at patients and the gruff tones used, even though the words themselves are harmless. Another common form of mistreatment is ignoring residents' calls for help (cf. Gubrium 1975: 156; Kayser-Jones 1990: 42). Confused residents who ask over and over to go to the bathroom are often ignored. Most aides screen out confused residents' incessant repetitions of words, phrases, questions, and complaints so that as one worker in Gubrium's (1975: 157) study said, "After a while you hear it so much that you don't hear it at all."

Aides frequently avoid eye contact with disoriented patients who sit in the halls and ask for help. This way they do not have to make excuses. When Mr. Hammond was brought back to his floor from the main dining room because his pants were accidentally drenched by a coffee spill, he waited in his wheelchair by the nursing station for almost half an hour to be changed. Deaf and extremely confused, he continually asked if he was wet, but none of the workers who passed even gave him a glance. When the nurse in charge finally asked his aide, Ms. Riley, to change him, she said she was too busy. Sometimes, aides stand by watching as patients struggle with enormous difficulty, and possibly some danger, to complete a task. Carmen Cruz, one of the few Puerto Rican residents,[4] was clearly having trouble positioning her wheelchair in her room. She bumped against her bed and chest of drawers as she pushed her wheelchair this way and that and even, in one move, hurt her hand. Instead of helping, Ms. Riley sat in a chair in the room doing her paperwork. Indeed, she loudly complained, "Why she keep banging up the place?"

Aides are sometimes insensitive to the residents' right to privacy. In her study of a California nursing home, Kayser-Jones (1990: 47) observed many dehumanizing experiences in which privacy was violated: "exposing patients' genitals, bathing men and women simultaneously in the same shower room, and creating a situation in which the elderly, owing to lack of help and attention, defecate and urinate on the floor." On any given day, Kayser-Jones says, one could walk down the hallway and see patients sitting in chairs or lying in bed unclothed. Rules at the Crescent Nursing Home eliminated some of these problems. The "no changing or dressing residents in the hallway" rule was strictly enforced. Residents were always clothed or covered in the halls or other public areas. Patients were wrapped in a bath blanket when wheeled to and from the bath; men and women were bathed and showered separately. Nearly all patients wore incontinence briefs, and there were no incidents, like the one Kayser-Jones describes, in which residents regularly urinated on the hall floors.

In the rooms, aides were supposed to draw bedside curtains when they changed or dressed residents, but only the most conscientious consistently did this. Many times, I walked into a room to see patients lying naked while an aide washed them. Generally, aides are more diligent about using curtains with alert residents, but even then, the mentally competent were sometimes left exposed while an aide did her job.

Disregard for the patients' sensitivities were evident, too, in the way aides commonly used residents' televisions or other possessions without asking. The severely demented were probably unaware of such behavior. Alert residents often minded. Jack Pollisi, a man in his mid-sixties, suffered from severe physical ailments but was mentally alert and had a wonderful wry sense of humor. Aides, he complained, would just come into residents' rooms and turn the television on to whatever program they wanted. "One night, in the ninth inning of a tied baseball game, an aide came in and turned the channel. I told her, you got to be kidding. I'm not one of your senile patients. And she changed it back." Another resident blanched but said nothing when Ms. Riley walked into her room to talk to a co-worker. Without asking, Ms. Riley took the resident's calendar off the wall and left the room with it to check dates for her vacation.

Perhaps just as bad as yelling and screaming are indifference and apathy—doing tasks with little energy or affect and not speaking to residents when providing care. One observer ascribes such behavior to physical and emotional exhaustion caused by job stress, or burnout, as it is often called (Heine 1986). A few Crescent day shift aides usually performed their jobs as if everything was a bother, in a sullen and distracted manner. One morning, for example, Françoise Bizet, a Haitian aide, was especially tired.[5] Overwhelmed with work, she had been unable to even squeeze in a few minutes for a break. She changed patients' beds in a hurried, distracted way, barely talking to them and muttering to herself about how tired she was. When she got to Mr. Gallo, she virtually threw a shirt on him, not even noticing, or caring, that it was wrinkled, torn, and the wrong size. Other aides who were generally friendly and supportive to residents sometimes had short lapses when they were exhausted or upset and did not focus on their patients or the job.

WORKER-PATIENT OPPOSITION

The pressures and abuse from patients in many ways pit aides against patients, so that we can speak in some sense of a worker-patient opposition in the nursing home. Residents have their own hostilities toward aides, of course. An articulate former high school teacher, suffering from, among other things, cancer and spinal ailments, complained that some aides were unresponsive, curt, and taciturn. Another resident made a thumbs-down gesture when her aide left the room, and one man, though often confused, told me, "Some of them are mean, very mean, and when you tell them, they're even meaner." Since my focus is on aides, it is their perspective that is stressed here. From their vantage point, the opposition with residents is fueled and reinforced by the institution's focus on patient problems and rights as well as by racial cleavages.

An incident that occurred on the second day of my fieldwork symbolizes the opposition in stark terms. I was waiting to get into the elevator with Doris Taylor, a black American replacement aide. When the elevator arrived, an ambulatory resident had some difficulty getting out. Doris did not immediately offer any help; the resident eyed her sharply and loudly proclaimed, "Another one of *them*." Doris offered a hand and as the elevator door closed, turned to me: "One of them! They're all like that."

As I later learned, this resident was famous at Crescent for her virulent hostility to workers and for her racist remarks. Yet, as Doris's comment suggests, patients, for most aides, are frequently "the other." Many aides do sympathize and develop close relationships with individual residents. But for the vast majority of aides, patients' demands and abuse, their favored status with administrators, their ability to make life difficult for aides, and their race put them, as a group, in an opposite camp.

Aides operate in an environment in which the focus and sympathy of the administration, government regulators, and the public at large are with the problems of frail elderly residents, not the workers. Aides feel that the administration overlooks their needs while pandering to those of the residents. When a severe hurricane devastated Jamaica, several Jamaican workers complained of the administration's lack of concern. "You think any of them ask how your relatives are in Jamaica after the hurricane? Do you think they care? Do you think they even think to set up some kind of fund to help people in Jamaica with clothes?" In a telling comment, one worker added, "They would say you should give clothes to the patients." In other words, patients' needs come first, with workers left behind. Administrators and professional staff make a point of knowing who residents are and going out of their way to greet them by name. By contrast, they usually ignore most nursing aides as they walk through the halls and rarely say hello.

Obviously, administrators are concerned with the residents' health—the institution is run with this purpose in mind—but aides often feel their own health problems are ignored. "You're not supposed to come to work with flu," said one aide, "but patients give the flu to you." Many workers, in fact, suffer from back ailments, and a high percentage have serious hypertension.

Administrative goals and government regulations stress patient rights and abuse. A twenty-one-item list of patient rights, signed by every resident, guardian, next of kin, or sponsoring agency, guarantees (at least on paper) freedom from mental and physical abuse and the right to privacy. Residents, the declaration states, "will not be required to perform services . . . that are not included for therapeutic purposes in their plans of care." Aides dislike the patients' right to refuse baths and other personal care, feeling it infringes on their own right to a safe, healthy, and hospitable work environment. "I'm the one dealing with the patient if any germs left there," one worker said. And aides worry about getting into trouble for abuse. "They're always coming up with patient rights, patient this or that," one Jamaican aide said. "Patient not even allowed to bruise himself without you getting held responsible. It's not fair. A lot of them have Alzheimer's and they hurt themselves."

While the administration and state regulators closely monitor possible physical abuse of patients, worker abuse goes unrecorded and largely unrecognized. "At meetings, they explain patients' rights, but what about workers' rights?" Ms. McKenzie, a Jamaican aide, said. "They scratch you, bite you. And you have no rights. All you hear about is patients' rights." Ms. Riley evoked gales of laughter from her Jamaican co-workers one lunchtime when she joked that she would run into the dayroom and lock the door if Dottie, a resident known for her violent behavior, came after her. Ms. Riley was not joking, however, when she added, for my benefit, "Cause you can't hit a patient back and if you say anything [report patients' abusive behavior] they [the patient] say you was the one who caused it."

Ms. Riley's fear of being reported by patients is shared by many aides. In truth, patients rarely complain about aides to higher-level staff. They fear reprisals. And they have little hope that complaining will lead to changes. Whatever the actual frequency of complaints, aides feel that patients have the power to get them in trouble. One afternoon, Nina was changing a confused resident who babbled incoherently. Suddenly, when Nina began to wash the woman's vaginal area, she screamed out, "Don't hit me, don't hit me." Nina tried to calm down the resident, gently reassuring her that she was not hitting her. To me, Nina added, "See how we can get into trouble."

Racial differences magnify the opposition with patients. Minority aides, who suffer racial discrimination and prejudice outside of work on account of their skin color, have to cater to the needs of and swallow abuse from the patients, almost all of whom are white. "When the patient call you nigger, you can't say anything, have to be deaf," a Jamaican aide told me. Moreover, most of the top administrators, who are viewed as the patients' champions and as unconcerned with the aides' needs, are white.

Although the racial gulf between aides and patients heightens the aides' sense that patients, as a group, are in an opposite camp, as far as I could tell, race had little, if any, effect on actual patient care in individual cases. These comments must, of necessity, be tentative as there were not enough minority patients at Crescent to provide a systematic comparison. Because of language problems, nurses tried to assign Hispanic patients to a Hispanic aide, and in a few cases, black workers had a black patient. From my observations, racial and ethnic similarity between patients and aides did not lead to better relations with patients or more sympathetic care. Interestingly, hardly any of the black or Hispanic patients were the aides' special favorites.

The patient-worker opposition put informal pressure on me to "take sides" with nursing aides and on a number of occasions created ethical dilemmas. My acceptance among workers hinged partly on allying myself with them, rather than with patients, and not criticizing the aides' behavior or interfering with their job.

From the very beginning, I was concerned that aides accept my presence and my role, agree to talk to me, and allow me to watch them work. Some initially suspected I was an administration spy. A few continued to be wary throughout my stay. I tried to dispel the aides' fears in various ways: talking to them and explaining my research; being introduced and endorsed by popular union delegates; even giving copies of my book on rural Jamaica to several Jamaicans to prove my academic credentials. I avoided spending time with administrators. I ate meals and took breaks with aides. On the floors, I spent most of my time helping, talking to, and sympathizing with aides and nurses. Although I became close to some patients, it was clear that to ally myself strongly with residents—and certainly to become an advocate for them and their interests with nursing staff—would endanger my relationship with many aides.

What was most difficult was having to silently watch as aides mistreated residents. Barbara Bowers and Marion Becker (1989), who also studied nursing assistants, mention the same problem of having to refrain from reporting workers and even feeling as though they were accomplices in poor quality care to maintain workers' trust. In my first few days in the nursing home, I was even reluctant to volunteer to wheel residents who kept asking to be moved because I worried this would get me into trouble with the nursing staff. Later, when I was more secure in my status, if a resident was stranded and there was something I could do, I would often ask a nurse if I could help out.

Still, I was always careful not to appear to criticize aides or to make more work for them. This meant that I did not interfere with or report abusive behavior. At times, I was deeply upset with myself for remaining silent without at least trying to stop or mitigate the effects of abuse by aides. I questioned whether it was morally right to place a higher value on the ability to continue research than on the patients' right to decent treatment. What upset me most were several lunches I had in the main dining room during which I sat with a couple of aides who loudly teased and baited helpless residents. They burst into peals of laughter as they joked about residents' quirks and found it hilarious to see a resident cringe after one of their verbal assaults. My heart went out to the residents. At these moments, I hated the aides, whose friendship and confidence I was trying so hard to win. I was mortified to be sitting with them and upset that residents would think I approved of such behavior and shared the workers' feelings. Yet, for the sake of my study, I felt unable to comment or intervene; this surely would have alienated the aides and earned their wrath. After I could bear no more, I excused myself and slipped away.

GOOD TREATMENT: KINDNESS AND CONCERN

"Life in the nursing home," Renée Shield (1988: 11) aptly notes, "is too complicated for exaggerated portrayals." There is a kinder and gentler side to nursing aides at Crescent than the one so far presented. In fact, most of the time, the overwhelming majority are considerate and decent caregivers. Of the thirty-five on-staff aides who worked on the day shift during my research, I would rank twelve as "excellent" or "very good" in terms of kindness and sensitivity to patients as well as conscientiousness. Another fifteen would be rated "good."

Personal styles vary, of course. Some aides are lively and chatty; others are quiet and soothing. Whatever their individual personalities, most are generally friendly and reassuring, and they listen and respond to patients in a kind or at least not unkind way. Often, they explain what they are doing when they touch or move patients and are helpful during mealtimes. Whereas Kayser-Jones (1990: 46) reports that personnel in the California facility she studied "stood silently in front of patients and hurriedly fed them," at the Crescent Nursing Home most workers talk to patients as they help them eat and tailor their feeding techniques to residents' needs. Most of the time, aides do not get angry. Dealing with difficult and abusive patients is part of the routine. Aides have come to know their patients' peculiar physical and mental problems, and they develop strategies to calm down agitated residents and get their work done.

Aides often try to reassure or distract patients when trouble arises. Nina Acosta, a friendly Dominican woman in her late twenties, constantly talked with residents as she worked. Brought to this country as a child, Nina had done nursing aide work since graduating from high school and had been at Crescent for almost five years. As she went from patient to patient, Nina kept up a steady stream of chatter, partly, I think, to liven up the job for herself but also to engage patients and get their cooperation. However provocative or nasty their remarks or abusive their behavior, Nina tried to be comforting. "I won't hurt you, you won't fall, hold on," she told a screaming and writhing Ms. Balsam over and over, eventually getting her to settle down. When a co-worker was at her wit's end, unable to position a resident who was scratching and yelling, Nina quieted the woman by kindly talking to her.

Other aides "work around" the patients' anger in different ways. Ms. Ross, a black American woman who had worked at Crescent for nearly twenty-five years, explained, "When they fight against you, I try to tell them something else is happening to get them to do what I want. It's a little white lie, but it seems to work." If all else fails, and residents continue in their abuse, most aides simply grit their teeth and carry on regardless.

Many aides actively encourage residents to become more independent. Self-interest is involved as patients who do more for themselves ultimately reduce the aides' work load and the physical strain of the job. Yet this kind of independence training takes time and patience. Nina worked hard to get Ms. David to eat by herself—"Before, she wouldn't do anything for herself"—offering continual praise and encouragement for her efforts. She also encouraged other residents to help wash themselves, turn, and sit up in their wheelchairs. Ms. McKenzie, an older Jamaican aide with a firm manner, worked to get Mr. Paul to help dress himself. "Lift your leg now . . . now raise your arm," she continually instructed him. She deliberately left the last button on his shirt undone, asking him to do it—"You can do it yourself"—and praised him when, after much difficulty, he succeeded.

Just as there are a few consistently cruel aides, so, too, a few never seemed to raise their voices and, as far as I could tell, were always gentle and affectionate. One of these four "saints" was Ms. Roy, a woman in her mid-thirties. A secretary in Guyana, she came to New York to join her husband, initially working as a live-in baby-sitter before training to become a nursing aide. When I came to Crescent, she had been there a little over four years. Ms. Roy knew more about residents' personal lives than any other worker I met; she often tried to understand their fears and anger in terms of their life histories. When she smiled to greet a resident and ask how they were, a real warmth came through. She carefully listened to and cared about what residents had to say and sincerely enjoyed it when they told her stories about their younger days. She never spoke to patients in a condescending way. And she did not recoil when they physically clung to her. "They need affection," she said. "I always touch patients. Yesterday, I was going to see Mr. Rose and I gave him a big hug and he just clung to me. Then he let go and we went walking and I said to myself, how long is it since that man hug somebody."

Ms. Roy took great pride in being close to her patients and was gratified that she could help people as part of her job. She once asked me how I liked Crescent. When I said I did but added that I thought, at first, that it would be depressing, Ms. Roy quickly retorted, "It's not depressing here, you can really help people." In fact, a great many aides spoke of the satisfaction they got from "making patients feel good" and taking good care of them.[6] Most aides like to see their patients look neat and clean, perhaps one reason so many enjoy giving baths. Like Nina, many take pride in "washing them good and thorough," and they worry that when they are off, replacement aides will not do a proper job. "When I go on vacation and come back," Nina told me, "I don't want to see anything. I take care of my patients good."

Many aides take pains to put attractive clothing and sometimes makeup and jewelry on residents[7] and are proud, too, that their rooms are well organized and clean. A number commandeered quilts from the nursing home's Christmas bazaar to decorate patients' beds. Ms. Ross put all the plants she had been given as presents by deceased residents' relatives in her rooms. She cared for the plants, which flourished. "They cheer up the room," she said. Aides take pride, as well, in their ability to cajole reluctant patients to eat. Ms. Wirth was gravely ill and lay in bed, motionless, all day; she had little energy or inclination to eat. Her aide, an older Dominican woman, proudly showed me how she mixed pureed food in a certain way so that "Ms. Wirth loves it; she eats everything."

Aides take pleasure, too, from feeling needed and becoming emotionally close to patients. "You're working here," one told me. "You're saving someone's life. They can't feed themselves, can't dress themselves. I feel I'm helping them." Quite a few used family images to describe relationships with patients. Some, after all, have looked after certain patients for years. When patients have no close relatives (or relatives who visit), aides often come to feel like surrogate family members. "You have to be there for them, like you're part of their family,"

Nina explained. "Put yourself in their position. Some of them have no family. Sometimes Mr. Schwartz, he will sit and cry for his son. His son don't come too often. I sit with him and tell him, 'Don't worry about it, I'm here.' "

As these comments indicate, aides frequently establish relations with individual residents that they and the residents find satisfying. Indeed, residents are sometimes deeply upset when their aide is away. One worker told me with pride that a patient would not take a shower until she returned from vacation. More serious, a senior staff member pointed out that another resident who was very attached to her aide had a serious psychotic episode when the aide went on vacation.

Inevitably, aides have their favorites, who may benefit from extra attention and affection. Other nursing home studies suggest that favored status and special care have a lot to do with the patients' ability to offer gifts and other resources to staff. The kind of reward most valued by Crescent aides—residents' concern and sympathy—has barely been noticed.

Drawing on exchange theory, Kayser-Jones (1990) argues that nursing home residents with resources are able to negotiate for special services and better care. An old woman in the California nursing home she studied mended and altered clothes for a nursing aide who, in turn, shopped for her. Another resident ensured that she had a steady flow of visits from staff by regularly handing out cookies and candy to those who stopped by. Patients can also offer psychic rewards in the form of "thank yous" and other expressions of gratitude (Kayser-Jones 1983). Thus one resident had few material resources but was well liked and given preferential treatment by staff because she never failed to express appreciation for even the smallest service.

Some Crescent patients did give aides small gifts of food and other items, but this, in itself, did not earn them favored status. Nor was it just a question of residents showing appreciation for aides' care, the type of psychic reward noted by Kayser-Jones (1983). What Crescent aides valued, above all, was patients who expressed an interest in and cared about them as people.[8] Again and again, aides told me and I observed that a resident was special to them because, as one worker said, "They show they care for you. They treat you like a human being, know you have a family." She went on, "They say, 'You work hard, you have to go home to your kids.' When they see you, they say, 'Hello Annie, how are the children?' " Another aide described her favorite patient: "Sometimes I come in the morning and she'll say

'Sonya, what's the matter, why don't you talk, what's wrong?' She notice my expression is different. If anything happen on the train (she hear it on TV) she say, 'I couldn't sleep worrying about you.' She ask about my kids. And when I go home I talk about her to my kids. I try my best for her. When she gonna die, I don't want to be there."

In their relations with most residents, aides are constantly on the giving end: meeting demands, offering support, and worrying about the residents' condition. Aides are sincerely moved when residents offer them comfort and are sympathetic to their needs. Maria Castillo, a young Dominican aide, was touched by Ms. West's concern that she worked too hard—"She say, 'Go home, put your feet up and relax' "—and her continual advice that Maria have more than one child. "Mr. Thomas," another aide said, "he worry about me. If it rain, he say did you get wet. He look to see if the train I take is working, he worry so much that I get to work safe. You know how it feel to have somebody care for you? If I fix his shirt, it's the same buttons I do, but he feel it's not like when anyone else do it."

Residents who express this kind of concern are among the more mentally alert. In fact, aides generally prefer patients who "have sense" at least some of the time and who understand what aides tell them. Workers also favor residents who do not complain or ask for too much (cf. Shield 1988; Gilliland and Brunton 1984). There were a few aides who found extremely dependent and helpless patients appealing, though often for different reasons. Ana Rivera, one of the "saints" at Crescent, had a special feeling for a semicomatose woman who lay in bed all day and needed total assistance. Ana's heart went out to the resident, who was alone in the world, with no living relatives. That the resident was totally reliant on her made Ana feel needed, useful, and important. In the case of Sybil Duncan, one of the facility's "monsters," her preference for two extremely dependent, mentally impaired, and difficult patients had different roots. She could completely dominate them. As she herself put it, "When I talk, they listen."

Abuse and harsh treatment are dramatic and sensational, but they should not obscure the fact that despite enormous frustrations and demands from patients, a great deal of sympathetic caring goes on at the Crescent Nursing Home. I am reminded of an afternoon when after unsuccessfully trying to feed a screaming resident, an aide in the sixth-floor dayroom threw up her hands in disgust and exclaimed, "This is a madhouse!" Yet at the same time, quietly and without fanfare, several co-workers kindly coaxed other equally difficult residents to eat.

This mixture of compassion and exasperation is a powerful reminder that aides' relations with patients cannot be reduced to simple all-or-nothing evaluations—and a reflection of the complex tangle of attachments, obligations, and antagonisms involved in nursing home care.

4

Institutional Demands: The "Iron Cage" of the Nursing Home

In his classic work on bureaucracy, Max Weber ([1947] 1964) writes of the inevitable tension between the demand for technical efficiency of administration, on the one hand, and the human values of spontaneity and autonomy, on the other. Indeed, the bureaucratic division of labor, in Weber's view, constitutes, in many ways, a "cage" in which modern men and women are compelled to live.

The tension Weber points to is clearly present at the Crescent Nursing Home and provides the framework for the analysis of institutional or administrative demands. Explicit organizational rules are necessary to prevent patient abuse and ensure decent care. Moreover, government regulations as well as the complexities of modern medical care require extensive bureaucratization. Yet, at the same time, the rules and procedures that have developed to regulate care are often a "cage" for nursing aides. They can discourage initiative and spontaneity and have some negative consequences for patients.

Another tension is built into the specific nature of nursing home bureaucracies, one that Weber did not consider. Nursing homes are institutions that aim, in a sense, to bureaucratize or rationalize affective care. Administrative rules regulate staff who, as part of their jobs, are expected to provide personal attention and sympathetic care to patients. Bureaucratic rules can come into conflict with workers' emotions and personal relations with patients, and patients are often the ones to suffer.

Bureaucracy's Contradictions

Some elaboration of these general comments will clarify the structural tensions or contradictions in the Crescent Nursing Home bureaucracy. What, to begin, are the pressures that push toward bureaucratization of complex organizations like nursing homes? Why are bureaucratic rules and regulations necessary in nursing homes? To Weber, who laid out the model of bureaucracy, the answer is that bureaucracy is technically superior to other types of organizations in coordinating complex administrative tasks. Its organizational efficiency, with a premium placed on precision, speed, expert control, and continuity, makes it indispensable in the modern world (Gerth and Mills 1958: 214). "However much people may complain about the 'evils' of bureaucracy," he wrote, "it would be a sheer illusion to think for a moment that continuous administrative work can be carried out in any field except by officials working in offices. The whole pattern of everyday life is cut to fit this framework" (Weber [1947] 1964: 337).

The superiority of bureaucracy in achieving coordination and control, in Weber's view, stems from its special features.[1] In defining the pure type of bureaucratic structure, Weber notes that organizational activities are carried out on a regular basis and constitute well-defined official duties, with each staff member having clearly demarcated powers. Staff, appointed according to technical qualifications and rewarded by regular salaries, are ranked in a hierarchical order: each official is accountable to a superior for her own as well as her subordinate's actions and decisions. The superior has the right to issue orders to subordinates, who, in turn, have the duty to obey—though the superior's authority is strictly circumscribed and confined to official matters.

Operations are governed by a system of abstract and impersonal rules applied consistently to particular cases. These explicit rules define the responsibilities of members of the organization and relationships among them. The rules are designed to ensure that tasks are done uniformly, at the right place and right time, regardless of who is performing them.

Aides may not be "officials" in an "administration" who apply rules impersonally, yet the nursing homes they work in are certainly highly bureaucratic. Indeed, nursing homes would be unthinkable without bureaucratic organization—not just in terms of administrative efficiency and to assure even minimal standards of care but to prevent serious patient abuse. Left to their own devices, there is no guarantee that aides would provide decent care. This is especially so given that many patients have serious medical needs and that aides have little, sometimes no, formal technical training. Unlike professionals, nursing aides do not come to the job having already internalized the complex rules, techniques, and standards of their specialty, inculcated through lengthy training (Perrow 1986). Furthermore, as one nursing specialist puts it, a nonprofessional health care worker performs her role "without a professional code of ethics to mandate and guide her actions, and without professional standards of practice generated by a professional organization and enforced in the courts of law" (Kjervik 1990: 201).

Nursing home aides cannot simply "do their own thing." The timing and procedures involved in changing patients and serving meals, to give just two examples, cannot be left to their discretion. While some undoubtedly would do a good job without formal rules and clearly-defined duties, many others would not. The horrors brought to light by the nursing home scandals of the 1970s—including patients left lying in their own excrement, scalded or even drowned in unattended bathtubs, and attacked by nursing home employees (Vladeck 1980)—would, in a rule-free environment, clearly multiply.

Indeed, the nursing home scandals led to stricter government regulation, and the regulatory process, as it has evolved, has been a major factor pressing nursing homes to design and enforce many rules and procedures in their facilities. Government bureaucracy, one can say, has bred further bureaucracy, encouraging and reinforcing an emphasis on formal directives and lines of command. Strict government regulation is absolutely essential to protect vulnerable residents from the perils of institutional living. It is all the more pressing given that many greedy providers would—and do—cut corners to save money and that some are simply cynical, indifferent, or callous about the treatment of elderly residents. In fact, since the nursing home scandals and implementation of tighter regulations, the most deplorable practices, though not eliminated, occur less frequently (Institute of Medicine 1986: 3).

Before a nursing home can receive Medicare and Medicaid funds, it must meet federal requirements; individual states are responsible for implementing federal regulations and for licensing and certifying nursing homes. The annual inspection, or survey, looms large. Until recently, surveys focused on a facility's organization: the physical environment, resident record system, and dietary routines thought necessary for a safe environment. Since the late 1980s, regulations have become tougher, emphasizing quality of care and quality of life as well as health and safety.

In New York, a weighty manual guides the inspection process, including instructions on meal observations and interviews with a sample of residents. Computerized data from the Patient Review Instrument (PRI) forms filled out for each resident every six months alert inspectors to possible care problems, for instance, a high rate of infections or use of restraints, that require on-site investigation. Whereas nursing homes used to know when they would be surveyed, now the visits are unannounced—"variable scheduling to promote unpredictability of surveillance," in the manual's jargon.

Though state inspectors only come to nursing homes on special occasions, government regulations permeate everyday work routines.[2] Certainly, this is true of the mounds of paperwork done, some in direct response to government rules, some a backup in case inspectors have questions about particular patient outcomes. Quite a few rules are in place and strictly enforced so that employees will pass muster at inspection time. No nursing home operator or administrator wants a bad report, particularly, Iris Freeman (1990: 297) notes, "as public policy moves toward full disclosure of surveys to help people make informed decisions about admissions." If deficiencies are found, this means orders for correction, reinspections to verify compliance, and, the ultimate nightmare, the threat of decertification. In unionized homes like Crescent, some rules are the hard-won result of contract negotiations, designed to protect and benefit workers themselves. These include complex disciplinary procedures management must follow as well as regulations concerning vacation days, leaves of absence, pay rates, and hours.

What all this points to is that bureaucracy, with its systematized rules of conduct, is, as Weber suggests, essential, desirable, and indeed inevitable in nursing home organization. But as Weber was also aware, bureaucracy creates certain problems and thus the tensions inherent in bureaucracy that are noted above.

As Weber saw it, the same features that make bureaucracy so efficient and able to coordinate large-scale administrative tasks also make it a monster. "The fate of the times," he lamented, is to live in a society characterized by "mechanized petrification." With its emphasis on strict adherence to rules and regulations, bureaucracy subverts the values of individuality, spontaneity, and autonomy. Modern men and women become confined in an iron cage or, in another of his images, like cogs in a machine (Giddens 1971: 216).

The ideal bureaucratic official does his or her job impartially and impersonally, treating clients alike and meting out equal justice in administration. These virtues, however, create "specialists without spirit" who carry out their duties "without hatred or passion, affection or enthusiasm" (Weber 1958, [1947] 1964: 340). Depersonalization is the outcome of bureaucracy. The calculability of decision making, Weber wrote, is more fully realized

> the more bureaucracy "depersonalizes" itself, i.e., the more completely it succeeds in achieving the exclusion of love, hatred and every purely personal, especially irrational and incalculable, feeling from the execution of official tasks. In place of the old-type ruler who is moved by sympathy, favor, grace and gratitude, modern culture requires for its sustaining external apparatus the emotionally detached, and hence rigorously "professional," expert. (Bendix 1960: 427)

Even then, the professional expert does not always make just decisions, and Weber acknowledged that bureaucracy may not deal well with some particular cases. A patrimonial ruler who delivers a verdict based on his personal knowledge of a defendant may reach a more just judgment than a modern judge whose mandate is to consider only the factual evidence presented.

Bureaucratic rules designed to make staff methodical and disciplined can, at the same time, encourage rigid and inflexible behavior—another drawback inherent in bureaucracy pointed out by Robert Merton (1957). Bureaucratic regulations can become an end in themselves so that employees simply follow the rules in an unthinking manner, whatever the circumstances. Because conformity to the rules is rewarded in bureaucratic organizations and deviations punished, the rules acquire a symbolic significance quite apart from their utility. Staff fear to take initiatives that violate regulations and proper procedures. Indeed, Merton (ibid., 201) argued that overconformity to the rules and the inability to readily adjust produce "timidity, conservatism, and technicism" and detract from organizational efficiency.

The stifling of autonomy and initiative, the tendency toward inflexibility and rigidity, and the encouragement of an impersonal approach to duties—all these, we shall see, are negative effects of rules and regulations for nursing aides at the Crescent Nursing Home. Yet, as in other human service organizations, the nursing home bureaucracy contains another crucial contradiction that classic theorists did not consider. Unlike the government bureaucracies Weber focused on, nursing homes cannot—indeed, do not want to—eliminate emotions. Whereas to Weber, effective bureaucracies manage to suppress the personal and emotional sentiments of staff as they carry out their official duties, nursing homes ideally provide affective care. The attempt to bureaucratize or rationalize affective care inevitably creates problems, and nursing aides are caught in the middle. They are expected and often sincerely want to be responsive to patients' individual needs and problems. But administrative rules can prevent them from offering this kind of supportive treatment. At the same time, nursing home administrators tend to overlook the expression of negative emotions toward patients. Aides who show anger and hostility to patients in their overzealous pursuit of efficiency are sometimes even rewarded.

In fact, the bureaucratization of nursing home care has had the effect of officially devaluing the supportive emotional labor nursing aides provide. As Diamond (1988: 48) notes, the emotional work of caring is an essential part of the nursing aide's job: "holding someone as they gasp for breath fearing it might be their last, . . . laughing with them so as to keep them alive, . . . helping them hold on to memories of the past while they try to maintain their sanity." Yet the bureaucratic demands of state regulation, pressures for administrative efficiency, and the sheer difficulty of formally regulating and measuring emotional care have conspired to create a situation in which aides are judged primarily in terms of the performance of physical tasks, which can be recorded in medical records, used for reimbursement purposes, and easily quantified. Caring for patients' psychological needs, which is not charted or paid for as a special service item, is missing from the usual litany of tasks and activities for which aides are responsible (Aroskar, Urv-Wong, and Kane 1990: 276; see also Diamond 1992). Indeed, as David Mechanic (1976, 1989) observes, medical bureaucracies of all kinds tend to give low priority to empathy for patients; they rarely reward staff who behave in a particularly humane way.

Other nursing home studies describe the limits bureaucratic routines place on residents' autonomy, dictating even their most basic activities: when and if they can be taken to the bathroom, put in bed, or bathed (e.g., Shield 1988: 188–190). The "tyranny of regulation" is how the authors of a collection on ethical dilemmas in nursing home life put it, as they recount the case of a resident forced to rise early each morning for a breakfast she prefers not to eat (Kane and Caplan 1990).[3] Likewise, in his model of total institutions, Erving Goffman

(1961) stresses the negative consequences of institutional rules and procedures for inmates rather than staff. In my analysis, the emphasis is on the way the nursing home bureaucracy regiments and restricts *workers*—and thus indirectly on how it impinges on the lives of the patients they care for.

The Hidden Injuries of Bureaucracy

The tensions inherent in the Crescent Nursing Home bureaucracy were apparent from the very beginning, in my first few weeks in the nursing home when I was assigned to one of the patient floors. In observing different aides on this floor and, later, nursing staff throughout the facility, it became clear that the very rules that protect patients and coordinate the complex aspects of care could also interfere with the aides' ability to provide compassionate and humane treatment.

It was the contrast in work styles of two nursing aides on the floor where I was first assigned—and the nursing coordinator's reaction to them—that initially made me sensitive to the hidden injuries of bureaucracy in the nursing home. Gloria James and Ana Rivera were exact opposites. Ms. James (as she was known) was cruel and abusive to patients, truly frightening at times in her anger and vicious behavior. Ana (as she was called) was gentle, considerate, and kind. Yet Ms. James was the nurses' favorite, while Ana was constantly criticized by the nursing coordinator in charge of the floor. Comparing the two highlights how kindness takes a back seat to the bureaucratic emphasis on speed and efficiency. Aides are encouraged to follow orders and finish tasks on schedule; they are castigated for spending too much time on "emotional work" with residents. Workers who take the initiative in trying to improve patient care and respond to patients' special needs can find themselves punished rather than rewarded.

GLORIA JAMES: THE FLOOR FAVORITE

Why was Ms. James so favored by the nurses? Mainly for being quick, efficient, and neat. Certainly, she knew the ropes. A black American woman in her late forties, she had worked at Crescent almost from the start ("I own a piece of the rock"), for twenty-five years. Nurses sometimes deferred to her expertise. When I was assigned to monitor residents' personal care items, both Ms. Gordon, the floor RN, and the director of nursing came to Ms. James to ask her where these items belonged. Ms. James was intelligent and a quick study, readily learning new tasks. A heavy-set woman with a loud, strident voice and sharp tongue, she was a definite presence on the floor, always ready with a joke or ironic comment.

Ms. James's rooms—"my office," she half-jokingly called them—were immaculate. By lunchtime, the beds were neatly made, with decorative embroidered blankets (that she had obtained) at the foot. Items in the drawers were properly in place and neatly folded. The yellow trays by the sink were sparkling, lined with paper towels to keep toothbrushes and other toilet articles clean. Ms. James was typically the first nursing aide in the dayroom at lunchtime getting residents ready to eat. She was a fast worker. She finished her "bed and body" work early and was punctilious about getting her paperwork done neatly and on time. When she returned from vacation, she was annoyed that her substitutes had not correctly filled out charts for the residents in her care.

Ms. James's attitude toward dressing, bathing, and feeding patients was much the same as her attitude toward her other chores. She was determined to get them all done quickly, whether patients liked it or not. Residents, in her view, had no choice but to take prescribed medicines, eat so they would not lose weight or be forced to go on tube feeding, or "do a BM" so they would not get impacted. She had no tolerance for patients' resistance, which slowed her down. Besides, she could get in trouble if, for example, their nails were not cut or their weights not done. In fact, Ms. James was proud that she could get patients to eat and "do a BM." I overheard her explain, indeed justify, her approach to one of the therapists: "Schmidt eats for me, but if anyone hears me they're gonna get me for patient abuse. I say 'You eat' and I'm a big woman and I have a loud voice. . . . Now Bernice Grossman, one day I was feeding her, saying 'Eat, if you don't eat, I'm gonna . . .' and her son, Dr. Grossman, was standing by the door the whole time and when I was done he say 'Thank you for getting my mother to eat.' She never ate like that before."

As these comments suggest, Ms. James's behavior to patients was far from gentle. Over and over, I saw her lash out at them. She bullied and taunted them; made fun of them; and even, on one occasion, almost caused a serious accident on account of her cruelty. Her tactics at meals were Gestapo-like: she badgered and yelled at residents in a terrifyingly angry voice. "I tell you EAT," she yelled at one woman in the dayroom. "You don't want to eat, you can die for all I care." When the woman meekly complained that she could not eat because her foot hurt, Ms. James screamed, "Shut up and eat you. Eat. You think I have all day for you." And she turned to another woman, "You're such a nasty pig. You hear me, drink."

When a resident Ms. James had put on the toilet complained, she barked, "Sit there. Just sit. I don't care what hurts, just sit there. Sit down, don't bother me about being ready." As the LPN passed, Ms. James loudly commented so that the residents could hear: "Two dingbats I got here. One has shit coming out of her ass and the other one says her back hurts."

Another time, well away from the nurses' view, she roughly heaved Ms. Schmidt out of bed and, as a joke, left her in a chair, unsupported and in an awkward position. Only the intervention of another aide, who helped position Ms. Schmidt in the chair, prevented a possible fall. Ms. James continued to verbally assault the sleepy Ms. Schmidt as she combed her hair. "Where you been last night Schmidt?" she taunted. "You been out on the town? Where you been?" When Ms. Schmidt replied that she was sleeping, Ms. James barked, "You must have been doing something, all you doing is sleeping now. You a pain in the butt."

Residents were not safe from her off the floor either. She particularly disliked Evelyn Frank, a woman with memory deficits, well known in the home for constantly thinking she had lost her cigarettes (they often turned out to be in her purse) and for collecting various inappropriate items in her wheelchair. She also often refused to bathe, a patient right that Ms. James detested. One afternoon, Ms. Frank wheeled into the main dining room where Ms. James was eating lunch. In a loud voice, directed at her tablemates but clearly meant for Ms. Frank to overhear, Ms. James said, "That is a dirty, *disgusting* woman. I wouldn't let her in my house. I would throw her out the window into the garbage or tie her up and throw her off the George Washington Bridge." She glared at Ms. Frank as she continued, "See how her tray so disgusting."

Ms. James humiliated and verbally abused patients out in the open: in front of nurses, administrators, doctors, and visitors. Yet she received the best evaluation on the floor and had privileges denied other aides. Indeed, when the two nurses were away from the floor, it was Ms. James whom they left in charge.

ANA RIVERA: BUREAUCRACY'S VICTIM

While Ms. James could do no wrong, nothing Ana did seemed to satisfy Ms. Gordon, the coordinating nurse on the floor. It counted for little that she was warm, considerate, and emotionally involved with patients—in my view, one of the best nursing aides in the home and the one I would pick if I were a resident there. What annoyed Ms. Gordon was that Ana was relatively slow and that she often ignored bureaucratic rules and procedures.

Ana is an expert in what Diamond (1988) calls the emotional work of caring: holding, cuddling, calming, and grieving. My first view of Ana was typical. As Ms. James and another "monsterlike" aide yelled at residents and bantered among themselves in the dayroom during lunch, Ana quietly fed a frail and weak resident, cradling her with one arm and gently calling her "Mama" as she coaxed her to eat. A woman in her late forties of Puerto Rican descent, Ana had come to the United States as a small child. When I met her, she had been working at Crescent for nearly five years, much of it on the night shift.

Ana was deeply attached to residents in her section and cared for them in a soothing and respectful way. I never heard her yell or lose her patience with a resident, even when she was suffering with one of her many migraine headaches or when residents whined, screamed, or were physically violent. In contrast to Ms. James's approach, Ana gently urged patients who refused to eat and gave positive reinforcement whenever they took a bite: "Good, eat, eat, it's good for you." Rather than rush slow eaters, she patiently encouraged them to take their time.

One of her residents, Ms. Calhoun, was a witty, sarcastic woman with Parkinson's disease whose mental status, as the problem book noted, fluctuated from alert and oriented to disruptive and verbally abusive. One afternoon she went out of control, screaming and shaking when a new rehabilitation aide mistakenly put a restraint on her chair. Ana gently removed the restraint and stroked Ms. Calhoun's head for several minutes as she calmed her down. "She [the rehabilitation aide] didn't know, it's her first time," she tried to explain to Ms. Calhoun. "Calm down now, calm down. . . . You're better now." (Earlier in my research, Ms. Calhoun went into a similar state when she saw a staff member cleaning her roommate's closet. She believed—and, given the frequency of theft in the nursing home, not without reason—that he was stealing her clothes. Ana was off for the day. The

LPN gave Ms. Calhoun a sedative when she started to get out of control, saying that otherwise she would scream and shake all day.)

With completely disoriented and unresponsive patients, Ana assumed a maternal air; with the alert, she chatted and joked as an equal, asking them what they wanted to wear, explaining the tasks she was doing or was about to do, and trying to reassure them about anxieties they had. One morning Ms. Calhoun was quite disoriented, yet Ana still tried to involve her in choosing clothes, asking, "What do you want to wear today? You pick." When Ms. Calhoun did not respond, Ana selected a dress a daughter-in-law had recently brought; she was able to involve Ms. Calhoun in a discussion about the style of the dress and whether the buttons went in the back or front.

Ana was one of the few aides I ever heard say thank you to a resident, and she did it often. One example: Ms. Calhoun regularly asked to be taken to the bathroom three or four times a day, something that Ana admitted made her job very difficult, although she did not show her irritation. One afternoon Ms. Calhoun made one of her many bathroom requests. Most other aides would have ignored the plea or stalled by saying they would do it later. Ana was much more considerate. Although she said, "I'm busy," she asked Ms. Calhoun if she could wait a minute. When Ms. Calhoun agreed, Ana replied, "Thank you." And she returned to take her to the bathroom in a short while.

Another seemingly slight but telling example of Ana's consideration occurred when I visited the nursing home several months after my research officially ended. I found Ana caring for Ms. Knight, a black American former nurse who, though a stroke victim and suffering from psychotic depression, was usually alert enough to engage in lively conversations. Ms. Knight took an interest in Ana's children and personal problems, and the two had established an easygoing, friendly relationship. I was glad to see Ana. We kissed hello, and I asked her how she was. Other workers would have answered immediately, and the two of us would have chatted, ignoring the residents in the room. Not Ana. Thinking of Ms. Knight's feelings, she said, before responding, "Say hello to Ms. Knight."

Ana empathized with the residents' situation and was aware of their family and personal histories. "It's not just a job," she explained. "Some of them are lonely. They have nobody; they need love and understanding." Ana's own mother died when she was six months old, and she was raised by her sister and brother. At work, she told me, "I feel like I'm caring for my own mother." She cringed when Ms. James screamed at residents. "It really hurt me. This place is like a House of Pain." Beyond emotion work, Ana was fastidious about keeping residents clean. She was careful about the way she gave baths and made sure to wash and lubricate incontinent residents when changing their undergarments.

But, as I have already indicated, her efforts were unappreciated by the coordinating nurse on the floor. One day she was berated for not doing certain tasks in the right order; another, for not having a resident dressed on time for lunch. If something was out of place in the nursing station, Ana was blamed.

Slowness was part of the problem. Though Ana maintained a steady, even pace throughout the day, she was sometimes late completing her tasks. Often, she was the last one in the dayroom at lunchtime; she was sometimes behind schedule weighing patients; and she did not always have her paperwork finished on time. Sometimes, she ended up staying late just to complete her basic chores. Unlike Ms. James, Ana was unwilling to sacrifice quality care for speed. "They say I take too long," she told me. "These are old people, you can't rush them through, shove them this way and that to wash them. You have to be careful when you move them."

One patient who slowed her down was Ms. Knight. Not only was she a "deadweight" who could not move any of her limbs but she had detailed requests and instructions about applying her "makeup, powder, and cream." Ana understood how important Ms. Knight's appearance was to her and willingly put in the time to "make her look nice." The coordinating nurse disagreed with this approach. She suggested that Ana cut back on her attentions to Ms. Knight to save time. The nurse was also concerned that Ana was spoiling Ms. Knight: getting her used to a higher standard of care than was required of workers. With her expectations raised, Ms. Knight would be upset when replacement aides (filling in on Ana's days off and vacations) cared for her. In Ana's words, "Ms. Gordon say I give too much attention to Knight. When you're not here, she say, how they gonna manage? She want makeup, Ms. Gordon say, she expect to be fixed up the way you fix her and when she's not, she gets angry."

Ana was unwilling to rush patients or deny them the small attentions that would make their life a little less unbearable. "I wish my job was easier sometimes, but I don't want to make it easier the wrong way, you understand." She was proud of the way her patients looked—

"Just smell them, you will see I take care of them"—and she wished she had more time to talk to them, to take them to the park in the summer, "to be able to really give them the care they need."

It is more than speed that was an issue with the coordinating nurse. I think the nurse felt that Ana was, in a sense, a subversive, undermining the bureaucratic order she worked so hard to establish. Ana was not verbally confrontational. Indeed, she was meek and apologetic in response to the nurse's criticisms. But by placing the residents' sensitivities and feelings before efficiency, she was, in effect, challenging the standards of her supervisor, the archetypal bureaucratic nurse for whom efficiency was all. If the rule stated that patients must be dressed and in the dayroom by 11:45, then the nurse expected them to be there, even if this meant spending less time on such things as makeup. Ana's failing to get tasks done on time, in fact, reflected badly on the coordinating nurse; if administrators came to the floor, she could get in trouble if aides were behind schedule and residents not ready for activities.

A major blowup occurred in the middle of my fieldwork when Ana was caught violating bureaucratic procedures in an effort to help one of her patients. Nursing aides must strictly follow the care plan laid out by the coordinating nurse. If they have a suggestion about a change in routine, from the food the resident eats to the kind of chair she sits in, the request must go through the nurse. As the professional expert, the nurse is the one who makes decisions about any changes and confers with other departments when necessary. New instructions are written on the care plan to guarantee medically sound and consistent treatment: the instructions are to be followed by workers on all three shifts.

Ana did initially try to go through the coordinating nurse to get a new kind of glovelike hand protector for Ms. Murray, a frail and partially comatose woman, who was one of Ana's favorites. The old gloves were not working, and it pained Ana to see the resident uncomfortable and vulnerable to injury. Yet after many requests, the coordinating nurse still did not order the new gloves. Unable to tolerate the inaction any longer, she took matters into her own hands and ordered the gloves herself. When the nurse found out, she was furious: "You cannot order things for the patient. You can only do what you see in the care plan or you will get in trouble. I have to write it down in the care plan, that is the only way to get things. You cannot do this. You are only here eight hours a day, five days a week. She is not your patient alone. The other shift will throw the glove away. You cannot be going around ordering things on your own."

The nurse's emphasis on bureaucratic rules and procedures was so overriding that she never asked why the new gloves were so important or what the problem was with the old ones—even when another aide chimed in, in Ana's defense, that the old gloves were no good. Indeed, the nurse summarily ordered the new gloves returned. More than a month after this incident, the nurse had still not even tried out a new type of glove; the old ones that Ana thought were inappropriate were still in use. Ana did not bring up the glove issue again, fearing it would simply get her into more trouble.

When the coordinating nurse blew up, Ana kept her peace, maintaining, as always, a deferential posture in public. In private, she fumed. The incident confirmed her belief that most nurses do not care about patients. "They should be glad I try to help the patient," she told me.

About a week earlier Ana was also reprimanded for going out of her way—and violating a rule—to help a resident. Rather than being praised for her compassion and initiative, she was punished. The rule was that wheelchair-bound residents could not leave the floor for an activity unless sent for or unless the nurse in charge approved and knew someone would bring them back. Ana was willing to ignore the rule to respond to a resident's plea. One morning, Ms. Knight repeatedly asked Ana if she could go downstairs to the main dining room. Pressed with her own work, Ana used her own free time, her morning break, to take Ms. Knight down. When she got back to the floor, the coordinating nurse attacked her: "You're not supposed to take her downstairs. Who will bring her back?" The nurse now had the added worry of having to make sure someone would bring Ms. Knight back to the floor. For the nurse, the rule ensured institutional efficiency, and it had to be obeyed. For Ana, the rule was constraining. If residents wanted to leave the floor, then they had a right to do so. "Is my patient, why should I refuse to take her? She feel lonely, depressed."

Ana was upset by the occasions when, out of fear of violating regulations and getting fired, she did not do as much as she could for residents or comply with their requests. There were times, she told me, when Ms. Knight looked tired and in pain. "She ask me to put her in bed and I say I can't, I'll get in trouble with Ms. Gordon. You're supposed to be dressed and ready for lunch."

Of course, not all compassionate aides run into the kind of difficulties Ana did; nor are cruel workers like Ms. James always rewarded. Efficiency is key. Workers who combine efficiency and kindness are well-liked by their supervisors; inefficient, sloppy, and abusive aides have trouble. And while workers who violate bureaucratic regulations to help residents always risk being chastised, much depends on how rigid their coordinating nurse is in adhering to the letter of the law and how effective in controlling aides on the floor. Two aides on another floor, for example, often bypassed their nurse in directly requesting equipment from the therapy department. Their coordinating nurse, poorly organized and lax in her supervision, looked the other way.

Ana's trouble, paradoxically, was that she had the misfortune to work on what the administration then judged to be the best floor, under the best registered nurse in the facility. In true Weberian bureaucratic tradition, "best" meant that the nurse was more organized than the others, always eager to systematize procedures. She exercised the kind of control the administration admired: she was firm in seeing that regulations designed to ensure efficiency and order were obeyed. That she was aloof and sometimes downright mean to residents—and indeed hard on Ana—were of no importance. In fact, during my fieldwork, this nurse was promoted to a higher-level administrative position in which she oversaw all the day shift nurses in the home.

At every level of the nursing department, efficiency and organization were valued over compassion to residents. An unhappy social worker was a minority of one in characterizing the director of nursing as a "caveman nurse" who emphasized efficiency at the expense of patients' quality of life. All the high-level administrators had nothing but praise for the nursing director's tough, hands-on leadership style and efforts to install systems to regularize procedures. It was the nursing director who initially assigned me to Ana's floor because she thought so well of the nurse in charge. I was advised to ignore another nurse altogether because, in the nursing director's view, she was so incompetent. As I saw it, this nurse, Ms. O'Brien, was wonderful: she was the most considerate and supportive at Crescent. Ms. O'Brien took the patients' complaints seriously, always tried to explain what she was doing, never in a condescending manner, and truly empathized with their position. Even when pressed with her own work, she always took time out to be helpful and kind. Her cardinal sin was having little tolerance for paperwork, although from what I could tell, she handled what she had to do adequately. Whatever her administrative failings, her warmth and consideration for residents went unappreciated by her superiors.

"Management On My Back": Oppressive Aspects of Bureaucracy

Ana's problem with the nursing home's bureaucratic rules was that they hampered her ability to offer what she felt was good care—a complaint shared by other especially compassionate workers. Compassionate or not, all nursing aides felt oppressed by the steady barrage of regulations that governed every aspect of their working lives.

What aides wear, when they can eat and take breaks, and what they do on the job are strictly defined. The care they give each patient is spelled out by the nurse, including whether to get patients out of bed, whether and how to apply restraints, when to give baths, and how often to take patients to the bathroom. As a reminder, a copy of the activities of daily living (ADL) routine for each resident is attached to the linen supply cart aides wheel around as they go from room to room. Aides, as we saw, are not supposed to deviate from these routines without the nurse's approval. The technical aspects of aides' tasks, from bed making to bath giving, are governed by definite procedures. Even patients' personal care items belong in specific places, something I knew only too well. At the nursing director's request, I was an unwitting agent of bureaucratic control. I spent over a month making lists and checking each room to ensure that such items as bath blankets and hairbrushes were in the right drawers.

What to the administration are essential requirements to guarantee efficiency and good care are from the aides' point of view oppressive regulations that crimp their style and limit their freedom. When I was at the Crescent Nursing Home, resentments ran especially high because, in an effort to upgrade the facility, the new administration was tightening enforcement of existing rules and adding new ones. A seemingly endless onslaught of new rules affected even the smallest details of working life. One day aides could wear jewelry to work; the next, after a memo went out, only watches, engagement and wedding rings, and small earrings were allowed (to prevent injuries to workers and patients). In response to a rise in theft, badges now had to be presented at the entrance to the facility, whereas before aides could simply walk right in. Suddenly, after putting lotion and shampoo in one drawer, they were told (by me!) to move these items to a different place (part of the attempt to systematize and monitor the placement of personal care items). "It's like a prison," one particularly disgruntled aide complained.

The new administration inherited a nursing home that in the words of one official, was "in the dumps," repeatedly cited for many deficiencies by state inspectors. The new administration sincerely wanted to improve the nursing home's departments and provide better care. Their own careers and prestige were on the line, linked to turning the nursing home around. The crucial measure was passing the state survey, which became a major administrative goal and dictated policy changes. A kind of battle mentality was associated with the survey, replete with preparedness drills and floor monitors who would go into action when inspectors came.[4] At the end of 1989, two and a half years after the new administrator took over, the home passed inspection with flying colors, with no deficiencies at all.

Aides were far less concerned with the state survey than high-level staff. To aides, state inspections simply meant that management stepped up its demands so that the nursing home (and administrators) would look good. Already, before the new administration came in, rules were in force which they heartily disliked. When I was there, aides were irritated by but resigned to rules stipulating how and when they did bed and body work, some of which they could and did circumvent. As in any organization, there was a disjunction between institutionalized rules and actual day-to-day work activities. Aides were on their own much of the time in patient rooms, and floor nurses did not strictly supervise the exact timing or performance of tasks like bathing, toileting, and dressing (see chap. 5). Despite my thorough checks, personal care items were often misplaced or missing altogether almost as soon as I finished my assignment. What especially annoyed and embittered aides were rules that were hard or impossible to get around and that infringed on what they felt were their personal rights and responsibilities or that jeopardized their jobs.

One gripe concerned limitations on telephone use: aides are not allowed to receive or make personal telephone calls on the job. Rarely are aides able to get away with making a call on the floor where they work, and even emergency calls are not supposed to be put through. The administration wants to keep the one telephone on each floor free for medical, administrative, and patient matters. On the give-them-an-inch-and-they'll-take-a-mile theory, there is a fear that if some personal calls are allowed, aides will overuse the privilege. Also, aides may neglect their duties and abandon patients to take personal calls. Such fears are not unfounded. On one occasion I saw a worker hurry to the telephone to receive a call (as it turned out, from her daughter's school), stranding a patient on her bed, naked, confused, and uncomfortable. Another aide made her priorities clear: "If a call come for me, I leave the patient on the bed."

From the aides' perspective, the inability to use the floor telephone is a hardship and a source of worry. Aides with families and young children are, in effect, incommunicado most of the time they are at work. A woman with a sick child must wait for her break to use the pay telephone on the main floor to check on her child's condition; her child, meanwhile, cannot call to ask her a question or tell her mother how she is doing.

Another complaint is the way the administration carps on and monitors attendance. Excessive absenteeism, construed as even a few days a month for several months, and excessive lateness, once a week or more, are common grounds for reprimands and disciplinary action. From the institution's and the patients' view, it is critical for aides to get to their posts on time. It is not just a question of getting behind schedule. Patients whose aide is late are forced to wait for help.

When I first came to Crescent, aides who clocked in more than six minutes late were subject to deductions from their pay. Still, there were problems. Many punched in on time but were late to their floor. The new nursing director issued one memo after another emphasizing the old rules and adding some new ones. When aides got to their floor, they now had to sign a daily staffing sheet; those more than fifteen minutes late were to be noted by the nurse on the unit. Aides who were not on duty half an hour after their shift began and who had not telephoned to say they would be late were to be replaced and sent home if they showed up. And aides were warned that if they punched in for each other, they would be subject to "immediate disciplinary measures." To many aides, these continuous memos and new regulations were another example of the "hassle they put you through" and the petty way administrators checked up on and restricted aides. "Like a slave camp," an especially unhappy aide said. "You can't be too late. Daley [the associate director of nursing] say you can't punch in without your uniform. The fear they have over you."

Aides who are out too often upset carefully worked out staffing schedules. Monthly staffing schedules are planned far in advance, and aides have to think ahead about when they want time off. Special requests for days off must be made at least a month in advance, and in March 1989, aides had to put in vacation requests for the next twelve-month period. Replacing aides who call in sick at the last minute is a nuisance. If the staff aide notifies the nursing home a few hours before her shift starts that she will be out, the fill-in aide from the replacement pool may not reach the nursing home until much later. This leaves many patients in the lurch and adds to the burden of workers on the job. A new rule was instituted to put peer pressure on aides to turn up by forcing co-workers to assume an absent aide's work load under certain circumstances. If an aide on the day shift called in sick, no replacement aide was now hired if there were at least three aides on her floor and there were fewer than thirty-eight patients. Younger women with small children generally had good attendance records. The pressure to come regularly was most difficult for some older workers, for whom the physical strains of the job were becoming too onerous.

The various regulations that monitor possible patient abuse are universally disliked and feared. Both the state and the nursing home want to prevent such abuse and weed out the perpetrators. Aides, we saw, are worried that patients will report them and that an innocent bruise may come back to haunt them. The required Accident/Incident form is particularly despised. Aides must fill out the form when, for example, a patient is hurt in an accident like a fall or when they observe a serious bruise or injury.

During my research, the nursing home called in the state to investigate every reported incident/accident rather than, as earlier, only when the nursing home could not determine what happened. From what I gathered, before I arrived, union representatives had instructed aides not to fill out the Accident/Incident form, in reaction to workers' fears that filling it out would put them in jeopardy. The nursing home, required by law to have written reports of abuse, mistreatment, or neglect, responded by informing aides of the law and appealing to the state to come in every time to make sure, as one administrator said, that "things are not swept under the rug" and, as another told me, that "we are covered when survey time comes."

Whenever an accident occurred—two broken fingers, one time—aides were abuzz with the news and sympathized with the worker who would be called in for interrogation by a visiting state inspector. Needless to say, workers did not like the accident/incident procedures. Superiors told them that the forms and investigations were not punitive but simply designed to pinpoint problems, yet aides who reported an incident worried they would be blamed and that their jobs were at risk. To be negligent in reporting was even worse. When the problem was discovered, they might be blamed for covering up. "Have you scared," said one aide. "If a patient have a blister you have to report it in case it becomes a sore. They make you crazy."

Aides were told about the purposes of the Accident/Incident forms at one of the many in-service sessions they had to attend, another bureaucratic requirement they resented. During my research, aides had to attend an average of three or four in-service sessions a month, each lasting about half an hour. Five of the "in-services" given annually—on fire safety, needs of the elderly, patients' rights, body mechanics, and infection control—are mandated by New York State. Others, on such topics as rehabilitation nursing, behavioral problems, and accidents and incidents, were designed by the nursing home to review and bring up to date the nursing aides' job skills and to teach them more about patients' special problems. Aides, administrators felt, needed retraining in even the most elementary tasks as well as instruction when added responsibilities, such as filling out a new form, were introduced.

Aides did not like in-services. In their view, the sessions taught things they already knew and did every day, interfered with getting their work done, and were boring. In-services run by outside experts were, in fact, generally uninteresting and unrelated to the needs of workers and residents. A sales representative for an infectious waste disposal company, for example, showed slides as he read, in a monotone, from company-prepared material that extolled the virtues of his firm. Another time, a company representative for mechanical lifts brought a videotape of a type of lift the facility did not own. He could not get the nursing home's lift to work, and a nursing aide had to take over and show him what to do. In-services run by the nursing home were better, but even most of these were fairly dull.

No matter how dull or engaging—and a few were quite lively, with aides participating in discussions—workers resent that the in-services interfere with their work routine and rhythm and make it hard to get their work done on time. One aide told me that in-services were the most difficult aspect of her job. "When you have too many meetings in a day, they take you from your direct work and take your time away from the patient and slow you up." In fact, conscientious and caring aides were often the most vocal in their resentment of in-services, for they wanted to spend their time doing a good job for their residents. Florence Wright explained how in-services disrupted her schedule and forced her to rush confused residents.

Say you have a patient who you put on the toilet every day at 2:00. They're confused when you get back from the in-service and say, "Where were you?" They get depressed when time pass on and I don't come. Now with an hour lost, I got to rush through my work. And, when I rush, I don't have the confidence that I do my job and have the time to take care. And when you rushing a patient, you're in a problem. They know it.

The nursing home administrator, a keen observer of his institution, was aware of the aides' grievances. Ideally, he told me, he would pay aides to stay for in-service training after working hours. He would hire lively, innovative instructors to stimulate and entertain workers and emphasize the personal and psychological aspects of care. Given financial constraints and institutional priorities, all these changes are unlikely to happen. As in place when I was at the Crescent Nursing Home, in-services were, to aides, simply another bureaucratic burden they had to bear.

The increasing bureaucratization and supervision of nursing aide work is a major reason old-timers look back to the 1960s and early 1970s as a kind of golden age. These were the days before tough state regulations were introduced, when the nursing home was privately owned and aides had a much freer hand in care. Despite the lower wages, heavier work load, and miserable patient conditions, many echoed Vanessa Bond's sentiments: "Everything was nice in those days."

Then, aides had more autonomy, less supervision, and fewer rules. Management was not, as aides now complain, "breathing down our necks if we don't get everything done on time." Strict schedules, endless forms, rigid rules—these were unheard of. They did not have to worry about patient rights or being reported for abuse. Aides could even use their own folk treatments on patients, like a brown sugar cure for bedsores that a few described to me.

Most readers will probably agree it is a good thing that aides can no longer improvise their own folk cures and that regulations to ensure efficiency and prevent patient abuse are in place, no matter how much aides dislike them. Yet to return to our major theme, what I have called the rationalization of affective care can, in certain ways, work against an important goal of the institution: to provide supportive treatment.

The sheer onslaught of rules has a numbing and demoralizing effect on the caregivers; it breeds cynicism about regulations and, for a few aides, contributes to a tendency to perform the job routinely and without feeling. Resentment of rules can spill over into relations with patients, as when workers take out their annoyances on those they care for. One especially bitter and rather cruel aide tried to explain it to me during an interview. "You writing now," she said. "If someone tells you don't dot the i, it would make you tense." She then spoke of the nursing home. "And who suffer? The patient. You scream at a patient. I could go in and see Catherine Murphy and smile and talk with her. If I'm under pressure, I not talking to her all day."

The steady stream of rules about and constant policing of lateness discourages the kind of commitment that management would like to see. Workers are loath to put in extra time, regardless of patients' needs. One administrator complained that he wished aides would stay back from lunch to feed patients or stay late to help nurses with hospital readmissions. A coordinating nurse told a group of her aides, "Yours is not an office job. You just can't take off and leave if it's 12:45 (lunchtime) if a patient is dying or if there is an emergency. Patients must be looked after." Aides are generally not moved by such arguments. If they are docked for clocking in more than six minutes late or reprimanded for returning late from lunch or a break, why should they stay late for no additional reward? Quitting time is sacred, and when the hour strikes, aides are gone. The next shift, in their view, can take over. Usually only slower workers skip breaks and cut lunches short so they can complete basic tasks—making beds, dressing residents, and giving baths—that, if undone, are easily spotted.

Conclusion

Weber's use of the image of the iron cage to describe the modern bureaucratic order is certainly apt in the nursing home context. The case material shows that bureaucratic rules, essential to guarantee the smooth functioning of nursing homes and patients' well-being, at the same time constrain nursing aides, sometimes in ways that actually work against patients' interests.

Crescent administrators sincerely want workers to be understanding, sympathetic, and compassionate—to treat patients, one told me, as they would their own mothers and fathers. Yet institutional pressures to provide competent and consistent care to frail, seriously ill residents have created a bureaucratic system that castigates a devoted worker like Ana and rewards a terror like Ms. James. Nursing aides who can be counted on to get the physical tasks of their job done with dispatch—and ensure that state inspections will be passed—are the backbone of the institution; those who are less concerned with deadlines and bureaucratic details and who ignore rules to help patients represent a threat to the institution's order.

The question arises as to whether it would be possible to allow nursing aides more autonomy without endangering patients' well-being and whether mechanisms could be introduced to provide legitimate channels for aides who feel blocked from being able to assist residents. I take up these topics in chapter 8. For now, I will explore further the tensions inherent in the nursing home bureaucracy by looking more closely at relations between aides and the nearest agents of bureaucratic control, nurses.

5

Supervisors and the Nursing Hierarchy

Relations with supervisory nurses are another source of pressure for nursing aides. It is nurses who announce and implement nearly all institutional demands, whatever their original source. Because nurses are the aides' immediate bosses and the direct enforcers of the facility's bureaucratic rules, conflicts are inevitable.

Too often, nursing home studies lump nursing staff together in discussing caregiving problems. This is a mistake. Nursing aides and floor nurses have different interests, responsibilities, and preoccupations and, often, different approaches to caring for the institution's elderly residents.

While much has been written about the hierarchical nature of physician (male)-nurse (female) relations in hospitals, there is little on women's authority over women in health care settings. The nursing home offers a dramatic case in which the limited role of physicians makes the dominance of female nurses over female nursing aides especially striking.

In hospitals, gender inequalities play a key role in nurses' subordination to doctors; until recently, virtually all physicians were male and all nurses female. "Handmaidens to physicians," "in the shadow of physicians and male-dominated hospitals," "victims of oppression"—these are some of the phrases used to capture nurses' low status (see Ashley 1976; Melosh 1982; Reeder and Mauksch 1979). As late as the 1950s, deference to physicians was a major dictum in nursing schools (Schwartz, de Wolf, and Skipper 1987). Even now, most physicians expect nurses to implement their medical directions without question and, at the same time, to catch their mistakes, like wrong dosages. In a well-known article, Leonard Stein (1967) details the subtleties of the "doctor-nurse game" in which nurses make it seem as if their recommendations are being initiated by the doctor. Even though nurses have more opportunity than doctors to observe and listen to patients, they must pretend that they never diagnose or initiate medical plans.

For nursing home aides, the key authority figures are nurses—not physicians, with whom they have practically no contact. Despite shared gender, a variant of the doctor-nurse game operates. Aides report observations of patients, which nurses incorporate into nursing notes, care plans, and questions for doctors. Crescent aides, unlike the nurses Stein describes, are free to put forward suggestions about patient care to nurses. But nurses are the ones who make decisions. Aides are expected to carry out the steady stream of nurses' orders, even when they differ over approaches to care, and to act in a deferential manner to supervisors.

Far from being romantic Florence Nightingales who gently minister to the sick and needy, nurses at the Crescent Nursing Home are preoccupied with bureaucratic requirements. As Rosabeth Moss Kanter (1977: 203) notes, nursing, like other female professions, features close supervisory hierarchies and concern with rules and regulations. Indeed, many Crescent nurses have much in common with Weber's ideal bureaucratic officials who carry out their duties with an impersonal spirit. Floor nurses devote large amounts of time to clerical tasks required by government regulations and internal organizational demands. Because they are responsible for what happens on their floors and blamed when problems are discovered, they are pressed to attend to supervisory details and infractions of rules.

The nurses' bureaucratic approach, to repeat a familiar theme, has limitations, and it places constraints on nursing aides, who are more personally involved with residents. Nurses can discourage humane and responsible care; some are even decidedly unsympathetic to patients. Aides who challenge a supervisory nurse's authority so as to help patients risk being hounded by her, as Ana, the conscientious aide, learned. Most aides would not get into trouble for a patient. They develop indirect strategies to avoid nurses' controls and let off steam by complaining to each other. Moreover, in a few cases, the nurse's leadership style tempers the effects of her authority, and although most nurses are women of color, race and ethnicity can also play a role.

The Nursing Hierarchy

Which nurses pressure and make demands on aides? During the day shift, the focus of this chapter, there are a good number. The director of nursing and her administrative staff, based in offices on the main floor, set rules and regulations, handle disciplinary measures and work schedules, and make spot-checks on patient floors. The nurses on each patient floor are also sources of endless directives. With one exception, there are two nurses per floor—the nursing care coordinator, who is a registered nurse, and the charge nurse, who is a licensed practical nurse. The exception is the sixth floor, which has three, an additional registered nurse at the start of my fieldwork, an extra practical nurse at the end (see table 2). (When I use the term "nurse," without any qualifiers, I am referring to both registered and practical nurses.) What the coordinating nurse says goes, and she has authority over the practical nurse as well as the aides on her floor. Each floor, in fact, is identified as "belonging" to a particular coordinating nurse. One floor, for example, is Ms. Vincent's, another Ms. Stewart's.

The practical nurse also oversees and assigns duties to aides, though she is a less awesome and more approachable figure than the coordinating nurse. She is closer to aides than the coordinating nurse in pay, educational level, and position in the nursing hierarchy. A few practical nurses, in fact, had risen from the ranks. One Haitian aide at the time I began my research was a practical nurse when I left, having finished her studies and obtained an LPN license. (Several Haitian women worked as nurses when I was at Crescent. Practical, as well as registered, nurses on the day shift were mainly Caribbean and Asian immigrants; several were black and white Americans, and there were a couple of Puerto Ricans.) Practical nurses spend more time than the coordinating nurses in patient rooms, as they give out medications, and they rely on the aides' help to change dressings and do other procedures. Although the practical nurse supervises the midday meal in the dayroom on each floor, she does not sit back and watch aides do

Table 2 *Nurses on Day Shift Duty*

Administrative Nurses (RNs)	
Director of nursing	
Associate director of nursing	
Gerontological nurse practitioner	
Floor Nurses	
2d–5th floors	1 nursing care coordinator (RN)
	1 LPN
6th floor	1 nursing care coordinator (RN)
	1 RN
	1 LPN

NOTE: The table refers to weekday staffing at the start of my fieldwork. (Typically, on weekends, only one administrative nurse was on duty, and one RN covered for all the floors.) By the end of my research, an LPN had replaced the additional registered nurse on the 6th floor. With the elimination of the associate director of nursing position, an administrative supervisor was added, as were four part-time administrative nurses who helped with weekend supervision and staff coordination.

their job, like the coordinating or administrative nurses who occasionally wander in to check. Her job is to feed patients, too, and in the process, she often chats and jokes with aides much like an equal. Off the floor, practical nurses and aides often eat together—several are regular lunch partners—and a few socialize outside the nursing home as well. It is highly unusual for a registered nurse to eat with an aide, and no registered nurses socialize with aides after work.

The high status and authority of registered nurses and their social distance from aides are symbolized in a number of ways that reinforce the nurses' position and enhance their aura of superiority. One such symbol is their uniform. Aides (and practical nurses) are subject to a strict dress code. They must wear white uniforms: an all-white dress or pantsuit (the most common outfit) or white pants or skirt with a colored or print top; white closed nursing shoes; and white or clear stockings. When I started my fieldwork, some aides wore comfortable white running shoes or sneakers, but a memo from the director of nursing a few months later decreed that no sneakers were allowed. Registered nurses are only required to put a white coat over their street clothes. And they can wear any shoes they choose, usually, it turns out, dark in color. Terms of address are also unequal. Aides always address registered nurses by the term "Ms." followed by their last name, for example, Ms. Gordon. Registered nurses, however, use less formal terms for aides. Generally, they address an aide by her first or last name, depending on what she is called by co-workers, for example, "Nina" or "Garcia," without the added "Ms."

On each floor, the nursing station is the preserve of nurses; aides are informally excluded. Set off by a 4-foot-high counter, the nursing station is the place where the coordinating nurse spends most of her time, doing paperwork; she is often joined by the practical nurse, also busy with charts and notes. The two chat with each other as well as with higher-level staff who come to look at patient records. Meanwhile, aides, on the outside, bustle back and forth, wheeling patients, carrying trays and linens, and rushing to make beds and dress patients. Aides rarely enter the nursing station itself, only going in for a specific purpose such as to get supplies from a cabinet. Typically, they stand outside, often leaning on the counter while they talk to a nurse or enter information in one of the record books. I can count on one hand the number of times I saw a day shift aide sit down in the nursing station. Only the boldest ever did so, and they were sure that the coordinating nurse was away for a long period and would not see them. The two chairs in the nursing station are reserved for the coordinating and practical nurses. (Symbolizing the physician's high rank, he always gets a chair, even if the practical nurse has to get up and stand; other professionals sit if a chair is empty.) Nurses and other professionals are allowed to make and receive outside calls on the nursing station telephone. For aides, this is strictly taboo. I witnessed only one aide who risked making an outside call when the nurses were off the floor, and she was on her way to being dismissed anyway.

Eating patterns, too, represent and fortify status differences between registered nurses and aides. Coordinating nurses do not, like administrative staff, have offices where they can eat in private. Nonetheless, they managed, during my fieldwork, to set themselves apart at lunch, in a closed-in conference area off the main patient dining room, where they could not be seen or heard by patients or lower-level staff. Aides, as well as coordinating nurses, seem to prefer this arrangement. "We should tell her she's not allowed to eat in here," Ms. Roberts muttered when her newly hired coordinating nurse seemed about to sit at her table in the staff dining room. Many aides, like Ms. Roberts, feel the coordinating nurse's presence would inhibit their conversation, and they do not want their superiors intruding on their own turf.

Nursing Aides Versus Nurses

The nurses' authority is keenly felt. According to the bureaucratic chain of command, floor nurses decide the aides' daily work assignments—when to take breaks and lunch hours, for example, and when to give patients their weekly bath. (Baths are tightly scheduled to ensure that patients are bathed regularly and that aides do not overlap in using the one whirlpool bath on each floor.) The coordinating nurse on each floor designs patient care plans and is the official conduit for requests for changes, a system that, from the administration's view, ensures consistent and professionally acceptable care. To aides, however, the need for nurses' approval for countless things is a source of continued frustration and resentment.

For example, aides cannot take a patient off the floor or alter care plans, even adding chair padding, without a nurse's okay. Patient requests often have to go through the coordinating nurse. Should a patient want to stay in bed, the coordinating nurse must grant permission. If a patient asks an aide for a certain kind of food, she cannot call the kitchen herself but must go through the coordinating nurse. The same is true if the aide thinks some aspect of care determined by another department needs changing, say, the type of chair used. Aides cannot approach other departments on their own; a nurse must do it. Because the coordinating nurses decide work schedules, aides have to go to them with requests for days off. When aides leave the floor—they are only supposed to leave for lunch, breaks, in-service training, or to transport a patient—they must let a nurse know when they leave and come back.

Aides are always looking over their shoulders to make sure the nursing coordinator or an administrative nurse is not around when they stop for a few minutes to talk with a co-worker or sit down in a patient's room. Sitting down and chatting are signs of loafing on the job (cf. Diamond 1988). Aides, administrators say, have plenty of time to talk to patients as they dress and change them. Afterward, they must move on to the next task. Needless to say, aides resent that nurses can sit and chat at the nursing station while they are castigated for similar behavior. Since the doors to patient rooms are supposed to be open, aides are nearly always visible from the hall. They never know when the coordinating nurse will be walking down the hall or called into a room, and administrative nurses deliberately make surprise visits to keep nurses—and aides—on their toes. If possible, aides alert each other to such visits. "Daley is on the floor checking the whirlpool," word went out one morning about the disliked and feared associate director of nursing.

Over the course of a day, coordinating nurses issue a steady stream of orders as particular patient needs and problems come up. "Move Turner," a nursing coordinator calls out to an aide, referring to a wheelchair-bound woman blocking the hall. "Bring Rosy back to her room." (Rosy Maggio is leaning over the nursing station counter, interfering with the nursing coordinator's work.) "Take Wright's weight," "Take Gross's temperature," "Help Hill [another aide] lift Jackson"—these are the kinds of commands emanating from the nursing station. "The nurses, they get on my nerves," complained a young Jamaican aide. "Because they're in a position and they boss you around, dump everything on you." Another described her supervisor in no uncertain terms: "a slave driver."

In her nursing home study, Shield (1988: 174) notes that residents tread a fine line: they must be persistent but not too demanding to get what they want and need. Nursing aides at Crescent face a similar dilemma when it comes to informing nurses of patients' symptoms. On the one hand, aides must report changes in a resident's physical condition so the coordinating nurse can decide on the appropriate course of action. Indeed, the new nursing administration constantly stresses how important it is for aides, as front-line caretakers, to report observations on the increasingly sick and volatile patient population. "You care for patients every day and can see if there are changes," a nursing administrator told aides at an in-service seminar. "You can catch pressure sores in their early stages or notice a problem before it becomes more serious." Aides who fail to make such reports can be blamed for negligence if a problem is eventually discovered.[1]

On the other hand, aides must avoid making nuisances of themselves. Under pressure to deal with mounds of paperwork, coordinating nurses have little patience with aides who interrupt them with too many questions or problems. A particularly testy nursing coordinator was deeply involved in writing up notes when Sonia Vega, a Dominican aide, approached the nursing station to report that a resident's foot looked much worse than usual. "Her foot bad, really bad. Can you come look?" Irritated by this intrusion, the nursing coordinator barked, "Does she have booties on?" When Sonia answered no, the nursing coordinator blew up: "Go get the booties. Jesus, can't you do your job? I'm very busy." The nursing coordinator did not bother to look at the foot or even consider a change in treatment. She was simply annoyed that she had been interrupted and that her care plan had not been followed. The aide was abashed and inwardly seethed. She certainly felt that after twenty-one years at Crescent (five more than the coordinating nurse) she could do her job and that she, too, was busy. Later, she shrugged off the incident as another example of the nurse's bad temper and lack of concern for patients. Next time, she might think twice about interrupting.

Even good-tempered and popular coordinating nurses are occasionally short with aides who continually bombard them with questions. Ms. Stewart sometimes lost her patience with a conscientious aide who was reluctant to make minor care decisions without the nurse's approval. The aide wanted Ms. Stewart to examine even the slightest change in a patient. One day, I heard Ms. Stewart gently lecture the aide, explaining that she should only come to her with important problems. "She keep running to me every minute," Ms. Stewart told me. "I can't do her job ***and*** mine, too."

Clearly, tensions between aides and nurses often have to do with their different perspectives on care as well as the structure of authority. Nurses tend to have a bureaucratic view and aides a more personalistic approach to patient care. As enforcers of the institution's rules, the nurses' first priority is that regulations are followed—that aides show up on time, adhere to care plans, complete tasks on schedule, and keep rooms and patients neat and clean. When nurses, on the floors and in the administration, check on aides, they are concerned with the physical aspects and mechanics of care: Is the bath on schedule and the whirlpool properly cleaned? Are patients' nails cut? Are patients positioned properly when fed?

As we have seen, the nursing administration and most floor nurses value efficiency over compassion. Slow but tenderhearted aides are criticized, while those who are neat and organized receive praise even if they are abusive. Admittedly, most aides take pride in their "bed and body work" and make special efforts to keep their rooms tidy and their patients clean and well groomed. But many are also concerned with their patients as people, and a handful are truly devoted in the attention they give.

Working with the same patients day after day, aides often become attached to many of them. These attachments can pit them against nurses. Some feel torn between the requirement to do their job with haste and the desire to spend more time talking to patients and seeing to their needs. Often, aides want to make their patients more comfortable when physical arrangements, such as chair padding, seem to be a problem and to help out when patients have special requests. Beyond altruistic motives, patients can become agitated and more of a problem for aides when their requests are not met.

Following proper procedures—and waiting for the nurse's approval or action on requests—usually means delays. When it is a matter of patient requests, it is the aides who have to explain the waits and comfort disappointed and frustrated patients. Mr. Schwartz wanted to use his money to order Chinese food for lunch, something he does a few times a month, which gives him enormous enjoyment. Nina, his aide, went to the coordinating nurse with the request. Busy with many other problems, the nurse forgot to put the order through. Mr. Schwartz kept asking where his food was, and Nina tried to explain the problem. "You keep pushing, pushing," she told me. "The nurse forgot, but I don't want to keep bothering her. She's busy. I feel sorry for Mr. Schwartz, poor guy. He really loves his Chinese food. I would go and get it myself—I did that once—but we are not allowed."

Taking matters into their own hands can lead to trouble, as when Ana bypassed the nursing coordinator and ordered equipment herself. Another time, Ana coached a patient to stand up for her rights with the coordinating nurse. Here the "getting out of bed" rule was at issue. To prevent a situation in which residents simply lie in bed undressed all day, the nursing home has decreed that residents, unless ill, must be dressed and out of bed by lunchtime. One morning, Ms. Knight complained to Ana that she felt ill—much the same as when she had a stroke—and wanted to stay in bed. The last time Ms. Knight made such a request, the nurse, a rigid adherent of rules and regulations, forced her to get up. Before calling the coordinating nurse, Ana told Ms. Knight that if she did not feel well, she should do what she wanted and stay in bed. True enough, when the coordinating nurse found Ms. Knight's temperature normal, she ordered her dressed and put in a wheelchair. Because Ms. Knight insisted on staying put, however, the nurse relented, saying she could remain in bed until the doctor had a look at her. Fearing that the nurse would suspect her role in this incident, Ana told me, "I'm gonna get fired from this place one of these days." Another aide, Ms. Braithwaite, an older Jamaican woman, felt sorry for and wanted to please a patient who kept asking for mint tea. When the incredulous coordinating nurse found out that Ms. Braithwaite had bought the tea for the patient—"How can she be so ignorant, you see what I have to deal with"—she was severely scolded for not first checking with the nurse to find out if the tea was appropriate for the patient's diet.

Quite apart from conflicts over patient requests, aides differ with nurses over the sheer enormity of their physical tasks and the time it takes to do them. Most nurses feel that aides have enough time to get their work done. It is just a matter of using it properly. Aides disagree. They have too much work, they say. One diligent and conscientious worker complained, "You cut corners because you can't do everything they assign you in one day." Another aide had an hour and a quarter after lunch before quitting time in which she had to give one bath, put two patients back to bed, change two, and do her paperwork. "I never have enough time to sit and talk with patients, always rushing. I guess that's how they want it." Most aides work hard to finish their beds, baths, and meal assignments and maintain a fairly steady pace throughout the day. Typically, they feel that nurses do not appreciate the physical and emotional strains of their job. When nurses, sitting comfortably at the nursing station, moan about their paperwork burden, aides have little sympathy.

Only a small minority of disaffected aides simply do not care whether patients are well looked after—including the physical aspects to which nurses attach so much importance—and take no pride in any feature of their work. These aides have nothing but disdain for the nurses' stress on order and efficiency and do the absolute minimum to get by and keep their jobs. They see no need to rush and push themselves for unaware and unappreciative patients who are near the end.

The majority of nurses are, themselves, far from ideal models of compassionate caring. Especially for registered nurses, the job itself encourages a kind of detached approach to clients that Weber saw as the mark of ideal bureaucratic officials. Involved with clerical tasks and supervisory details, these nurses spend little time with patients. Most registered nurses are cool, often aloof with patients as they plow ahead with their paperwork and other official duties.

Pressed to complete their own assigned work—and interrupted countless times by aides, patients, physicians, family members, and administrators—both registered and practical nurses on the floors sometimes take out their frustrations on defenseless residents. Nurses tolerate a high level of psychological abuse. The kind of patient abuse they worry about is physical; it may leave telltale signs that must be reported to the state. I never heard nurses talk with aides about how they should behave toward patients in psychological terms. Emotional abuse is ignored. Nurses who go out of their way to be kind and considerate to residents are a distinct minority. Only three of the twenty-four practical and registered nurses I closely observed were truly gentle in their approach; the one registered nurse among them was derided as inefficient by the nursing administration. A fourth nurse was concerned with and made arrangements to try to improve the patients' emotional states, though she herself was offhand with patients most of the time.

Nurses were sometimes cruel, occasionally quite vicious, toward patients. One afternoon I was in the nursing station on one floor, along with the physician, the coordinating nurse, and the dietitian. The coordinating nurse was busy organizing and writing down patient weights when Elsa Howard wheeled by crying, "Please, please, change me, I'm wet." The nurse dismissed this plea, telling her she had gone recently, that her aide, Ms. Hill, would soon be back from lunch, that she could not stay at the nursing station, and that someone would help her. A few minutes later, Ms. Howard returned. "Please help me, I'm wet already, I went wee wee in my pants. It will only take a minute." At this point, the coordinating nurse exploded: "This is not my job; it's the nurse's aide's job to change you." Well aware that Ms. Hill was still at lunch, she added, "Get Hill." When Ms. Howard said that she could not find Ms. Hill, the nurse yelled, "Go down the hall and make an aide do it. It takes more than a few minutes. I have my work to do." Embarrassed that I had overheard this exchange, the physician commented, "That's going to be some interesting book you write." The dietitian remarked, "That is how she [the coordinating nurse] gets her work done." Nurses typically ignore or belittle similar kinds of patient pleas, although some coordinating nurses would have been kinder and more diligent in getting an aide to change Ms. Howard.

Take another incident involving the model nursing coordinator, Ms. Gordon, who made fun of and deliberately lied to a patient, Evelyn Frank. Usually, Ms. Frank spent the day in the main floor dining room where she could smoke with impunity, but when the dining room was closed one day for a special activity, she was forced back onto her floor. Because in the past she had been caught smoking in her room, which is strictly taboo, the practical nurse had taken away her cigarettes. "I need a smoke," pleaded Ms. Frank, who was miserable, not having had a cigarette for hours. The nursing coordinator told her she could smoke in the dayroom, knowing full well that Ms. Frank's cigarettes had been confiscated. Given her memory lapses, normally Ms. Frank would have begun to search, with extreme agitation, for her cigarettes, but this time she remembered what had happened and complained, "They took my cigarettes from me." The nursing coordinator simply shrugged and looked over at the practical nurse. The two of them laughed, while Ms. Frank sat cowed and helpless.

I witnessed many other instances in which nurses berated, taunted, or made nasty comments to patients who violated floor rules or interrupted routines with complaints or problems. Simply ignoring a complaining resident, or shoving her wheelchair absentmindedly aside, was common. One belligerent practical nurse consistently bullied and made fun of patients. Her angry cursing and shouts of "shut up" and "stop it" continually rang through the halls.

Most aides shrug off nurses' callous treatment of patients as an inevitable part of nursing home life, and, of course, some engage in similar kinds of taunts and abuse themselves. Nurses' harsh behavior—an all too common feature of several floors—is, however, painful to the few especially compassionate aides who feel powerless in the face of their superiors' abuse.

Whether grievances against nurses stem from different approaches to care or the sheer weight of nurses' authority, aides frequently vent their anger by complaining to each other. An especially unpopular administrative nurse, Ms. Daley, was a constant topic of conversation, roundly cursed time after time. She need only cough in the staff dining room, and aides muttered among themselves about how she was polluting the food. Hispanic and Haitian aides can get away with direct verbal assaults in Spanish or Creole if the nurse in question does not speak the language. And English-speaking West Indians sometimes use patois to make nurses uncomfortable. "When me and Roberts are in the elevator with Marcos," a Jamaican aide told me about a Filipino nurse she detested, "we talk 'Jamaican' on purpose so she can't understand."

Despite their complaints, the fact is that aides are able to protect their work terrain from nurses' interference to a large extent. Usually, no one is watching while they care for patients. It is rare for a nurse to specifically come to check on them: coordinating nurses do not go out of their way to observe aides bathing, toileting, or dressing patients.

The nurses' philosophy is that if an aide is derelict in her duty, a problem will turn up, for example, a patient will develop a rash or look dirty. Although practical nurses observe aides as they move around the floor, they have a sense of camaraderie with aides. Practical nurses tend to be careful not to antagonize aides when they offer suggestions or criticisms. One administrator after another complained to me that coordinating nurses, who are supposed to be running the floors, do not have sufficient control. To increase coordinating nurses' vigilance and weaken aides' power, the director of nursing assigned an administrative nurse to work with the coordinating nurses, arranged a management course for nurses, and planned to rotate aides on the floors. When I did my research, nearly all staff aides were permanently assigned a section, with the exception of a few floaters who filled in for workers on their days off. Some aides had been working in the same rooms, and with many of the same patients, for years and felt proprietary over "their" section. By rotating aides among sections on a floor every few months, the director of nursing aimed to break them of the notion that they owned their sections and to make them easier to supervise.

In practice, aides are able to circumvent quite a few nursing directives. Care plans are not followed religiously. Even the most conscientious aides do not change patients or take them to the bathroom the requisite number of times.[2] Paperwork is often not done on schedule. For example, aides often fill in the accountability sheet the day after the tasks are actually done, automatically checking off what is expected. While aides are scrupulous about one-hour lunches—those on second lunch cannot leave the floor until the "first-lunchers" return—most are gone longer than fifteen minutes for the morning break. And while aides are not supposed to sit in patient rooms and chat with each other, when nursing coordinators are out of sight, they occasionally do so, especially on floors where the practical nurse looks the other way.

Aides are safe as long as they gossip out of the nurses' sight and are not caught violating the rules. To directly challenge a nursing coordinator's, or administrative nurse's, authority, particularly her medical orders, is risky, however. Generally, only the most secure dare to do so. Even then, they usually use oblique aggressive techniques. Aides who get on well with their coordinating nurses frequently engage in a joking relationship with them as a way to question orders and make their views known. By couching challenges in a teasing and joking manner, the seriousness of the intent is ambiguous (see Halle 1984). The coordinating nurse is able to laugh at the joking comments and not take offense. Ms. Hill gets on well with her coordinating nurse and is a trusted aide on her floor. One afternoon she asked the coordinating nurse to look at a patient she was weighing who seemed to have gained a lot of weight. When the supervisor said she did not have to look, Ms. Hill resorted to joking to get her way. "That lady heavy," Ms. Hill said, "and I'm not getting her on the scale again." The coordinating nurse smiled and got up. "OK, I'll have a look."

Another aide, Sybil Duncan, who was secure in her position owing to her important union role, adopted a different, more aggressive indirect strategy. Annoyed by her nursing coordinator's insistence on strictly abiding by the rules—"She used to be on my back"—Ms. Duncan took the nurse's policy to its logical extreme: "When I need a gown and she downstairs, I page her. When I need soap, I page her. Anything I want, anywhere she is, I page her till she get frustrated. As I see any little blotch, I call the nurse for my patient. I say you need to document it. I drive her crazy; I call her for every goddamn thing. When I done, she was a very nice supervisor. She been OK with me for a long time."

Most aides are not comfortable enough with their supervisors to take the license Ms. Hill did or sure enough of the invincibility of their position to dare a strategy like Ms. Duncan's. They fear the consequences—ultimately, their jobs—if they step out of line. Nursing coordinators have been known to "punish" insubordinate aides by going out of their way to criticize them for even slight deviations from procedures, a fate Ana suffered. "Put a whole strip of mess against you," is how one aide put it. Sometimes, nurses are particularly cool to a defiant aide. More serious, they may write a bad evaluation and set the stage for disciplinary measures. Ms. Riley's insolence was doubtless one factor in the lukewarm evaluation she received when I was around. One example: Told to straighten out her patients' drawers because of the upcoming state inspection, Ms. Riley defiantly told the coordinating nurse, "I will not do it. I have too much work to do."

Typically, aides are deferential in the face of their superior's criticisms, even when boiling inside. They do not challenge the legitimacy of the order or criticism itself, as Ms. Riley did. Rather, they shift the blame for the messy drawers, dirty nails, unmade bed, or other "misdemeanor" away from themselves. It is the fault of workers on another shift, aides commonly say, or workers who replaced them on their day off. In their defense, aides insist that they have too many patients and too little time to complete their work properly. As Margaret Lewis responded when the coordinating nurse criticized her sloppy work, "I have too much work to do now, and the other shift don't do nothing. It all fall on the day shift" (see Gubrium 1975: 147).

Popular and Unpopular Nurses

So far, one might expect aides to have nothing but resentment for their supervisors. In fact, this is not so. While some nurses are viewed with intense hostility, others, on the patient floors and in the administration, are well liked and immune to criticism.

Floor nurses, in particular, are what classic writers on organizations, before the days of feminist scholarship, called "men in the middle": they are caught between the demands of management, on the one hand, and the resistance of workers they supervise, on the other (Kanter 1977: 186–187). At the Crescent Nursing Home, management, from above, pressures nurses to supervise aides strictly so floors run smoothly, properly, and on schedule; while aides, from below, resent and resist nurses' authority and discipline. Whether or not nurses are popular with aides has a lot to do with how they handle their ambiguous position. In general, leadership style and, to a lesser extent, race and ethnicity determine whether structural inequalities and conflicting perspectives between nurses and aides lead to serious strains.

Which nurses are especially disliked? Essentially, those whose main orientation is to the management hierarchy and who make no, or few, attempts to curry favor with workers. Unpopular nurses generally have quick tempers, are unsympathetic to aides' problems, and act in a haughty manner. One unpopular coordinating nurse had two basic styles with aides: she made critical comments or maintained a cool distance. Another issued orders in a brusque, often distracted way. Inevitably, she barked at aides who disturbed her concentration on paperwork. Indeed, when I interrupted this nurse one day to ask a question, she began to yell at me. She quickly changed her tone, however, when she realized it was I who had bothered her and not an aide. A temporary agency nurse, around about a month, was roundly criticized by staff at all levels for her blunt, abrasive, and biting manner.

Aides are deeply sensitive to implications that they are inferior and unworthy of respect. Nurses who show disdain for aides and make no effort to establish friendly relations come under constant attack. One aide complained that Ms. Vincent says things like, "Did the troops get all my temps?" "You don't want anyone approach you like that," the aide explained, "call you the troops, instead of your name. Nobody like that." Another aide, on a different floor, had this to say about her coordinating nurse: "She thinks we just five girls and she a big responsible lady." Aides talk bitterly of supervisors who convey the impression that "dirtying their hands to help out" is beneath them. And there is a feeling, too, that some nurses have it in for members of particular ethnic groups. "Ms. Vincent, she don't like foreigners," said a West Indian of a black American nurse.

If ethnic differences accentuate tensions with inconsiderate or heavy-handed nurses, this is even more true of race. Most extreme was the intense hostility directed against the white American associate director of nursing, the model of an unpopular nurse. Ms. Daley's administrative role—as watchdog on the patient floors, disciplinarian of aides, and chief of scheduling—put her in a difficult position. On the floors, she had to issue orders and reprimand delinquent workers; in her office, she frequently had to deny aides' pleas for schedule changes and summon them to discuss disciplinary problems. Yet other nurses who assumed Ms. Daley's responsibilities after she left managed to establish much smoother relations with aides. It was largely a matter of personal style. Uninterested in gaining the aides' affection and intent on running a tight ship, Ms. Daley was authoritarian and condescending, and the aides both hated and feared her. The racial and cultural gap magnified her social distance from the aides.

"She gives orders like an admiral in the navy," is how one aide described Ms. Daley. This was not far from the truth. A big woman with a loud voice and rigid bearing, she issued commands in a cold peremptory manner. When an aide lowered her eyes as Ms. Daley was scolding her, Ms. Daley snapped, "Don't look away from me." A well-educated Jamaican aide, who had gone to college for one year, complained, "She treats you like a child. She talks to you like you're stupid. I refuse to let her talk to me like that, because I went to college. She likes to put people down." Aides resented that Ms. Daley often impugned their abilities, immediately assuming that they were not doing their job correctly as she made checks on the floors.

Unwilling or unable to couch her criticisms in a friendly and light manner, Ms. Daley's approach was typically cold and relentless. One example is an incident involving Ms. James, the floor favorite described previously. Ms. Daley was on the floor, at lunchtime, making one of her routine checks. Walking over to the nursing station, where Ms. James was chatting with a nurse, Ms. Daley addressed Ms. James in a schoolmarmish voice: "Ms. James, go look at Grossman and see if you notice anything." Abashed, Ms. James headed for the dayroom to check on Ms. Grossman. She soon returned to the nursing station, happy that she had discovered the problem. "I see," she said cheerily, "her nails need doing. I didn't have my clippers on me this morning. I'll cut Bernice's nails after lunch." Ms. James assumed the incident was over, but Ms. Daley sternly pressed on. "You could have gotten the scissors from the front desk."

Ms. James, who usually jokes with her superiors, was surprisingly deferential in this encounter. Indeed, most aides were intimidated by Ms. Daley. Workers were always "watching out for Daley." "I'll tell you if Daley coming," a shout went out to a co-worker who was writing up records in a patient's room. Many times aides complained about a task, for example, cleaning the whirlpool bath, but were pressed to do it anyway: "Daley says I have to."

I, too, assimilated the aides' attitudes toward Ms. Daley. For a long time, I viewed her as an intimidating ogre, whom I was reluctant to approach. When I finally went to see her, to ask for some statistics, I was surprised that she was warm and friendly and went out of her way to be helpful. This, I learned, was her general manner with those she deemed to be of similar or higher status. Although she subsequently made many friendly overtures to me, I was afraid to become too closely identified with her. On a number of occasions, she invited me to join her at lunch in the main dining room. Knowing the aides' eyes would be on me, I demurred, telling her that for my research I needed to eat with aides.

Much to the aides' relief, Ms. Daley was dismissed by the new director of nursing, Ms. Grant, several months after I arrived. Whether Ms. Daley's leadership style was a factor is unclear. More important was the director of nursing's desire for a loyal administrative staff. She had not hired Ms. Daley. And she was angered by Ms. Daley's insubordination, including complaints to the administrator. Interestingly, some aides interpreted the disagreement between Ms. Daley and Ms. Grant in racial terms. "Daley didn't want to work under a black woman," as one worker said.

Popular nurses at Crescent were, in fact, women of color. Race drew them closer to aides, and shared ethnicity could also reduce strains. The key to nurses' popularity, however, was the careful cultivation of good relations with workers—showing concern for aides' problems and taking time to chat and joke with them in a comradelike way, even as they issued instructions and made critiques. Indeed, two of the most well-liked and respected nurses, the director of nursing and Ms. Stewart, a coordinating nurse, were also among the strictest. They were able to introduce tougher regulations and more tightly structured regimes without arousing animosity because they were masters of interpersonal relations.

On the face of it, Ms. Grant had every reason to be despised. A newcomer, she launched a program of reform in her role as director of nursing which made life more difficult for aides. She sent out one unpopular memo after another, announcing, for example, tighter rules to stem lateness and absenteeism and stricter enforcement of the dress code. Aides bristled at each change, yet Ms. Grant herself was personally spared attack.

Partly, this had to do with the way she introduced major changes. After six months on the job, Ms. Grant decided to alter the shift hours. Rather than proceed arbitrarily, she slowly built up a consensus by holding meetings with union delegates and developing majority support for the change among aides on all three shifts. (Many day shift workers opposed the change, but they were outnumbered by aides on other shifts who welcomed the new hours.) After I left, Ms. Grant gradually introduced on-unit rotation of aides whereby aides on a floor changed sections (and patients) every six months or so. As she explained, "You cannot just come in one day and say to someone working with the same section for fifteen years, you are going to change tomorrow. There has to be preparation." On floors where aides were resistant to rotation, she held off, allowing the old system to remain while aides had time to adjust to the new concept.

While there was never any doubt that Ms. Grant was in charge, she did not emphasize her superior rank in exchanges with aides. She made it clear that menial tasks were not beneath her, and I occasionally saw her help out on the floors by taking a patient to the bathroom or lending a hand at meals. In general, she had an easy, relaxed manner with aides, joking with them and tossing off criticisms in a light, friendly, nonthreatening way. She sometimes lapsed into patois with Jamaican aides and, like other West Indians, frequently touched aides as she talked with them. Whether or not she was conscious of it, she sounded less West Indian and more "American" when she spoke with black Americans. Although swamped with work and rushed to meet deadlines and appointments, Ms. Grant talked to aides on the floors as if she had all the time in the world. She never appeared hurried, giving aides her full attention and patiently listening to their stories and problems. She was careful, too, not to antagonize senior aides in her effort to institute changes and often went out of her way to defer to their experience and expertise. When Ms. Grant was preparing a memo detailing how aides should organize patients' personal care items, she appealed to an old-timer: "I need you, you have to tell me where they [the toilet articles] go. I need your help on this, I don't want to make mistakes."

Ms. Stewart, a nursing coordinator on one of the floors, was another genius at leadership, able to assert control at the same time as she gained the loyalty of her staff. Like Ms. Grant, she was strict about enforcing many rules. Yet also like Ms. Grant, she was tactful and easygoing in her approach. New to the job, she deliberately tried to build up morale and gain the aides' trust so that she could institute major changes. She rotated aides several months before the official order went out, for example.

From her very first days at Crescent (she arrived a couple of months after I did), Ms. Stewart carefully nurtured good relations with her staff. She jokingly deferred to an older Jamaican aide, calling her "the general," and made a special effort to establish an alliance with another, potentially recalcitrant, Jamaican. Her usual manner with aides was to engage in constant banter, whether she was explaining rules, giving instructions, or, as often happened, holding forth on some issue like medical treatment or bureaucratic delays.

Like Ms. Grant, Ms. Stewart was a hands-on leader, not too "great" to help out with menial tasks. Without losing any of her forceful authority, she also developed a camaraderie with her staff. When she bought a soda, she offered to share it with aides; on several occasions, she ate with aides in the staff dining room; and she readily gossiped, shared stories, and laughed with them.

Ms. Stewart showed real empathy for the aides' difficulties, and she had a confident and maternal manner in dispensing advice. That she spoke Spanish (she was a West Indian from Central America) gave her a bond with the Dominican aides, and she shared a West Indian cultural style with the Jamaicans. (There were two Jamaicans, two Dominicans, and one black American permanently assigned to the floor, and another Jamaican and Dominican regularly filled in when needed.) I think aides appreciated that she was so solicitous of them, and they admired her as a model of a black immigrant professional. When Ms. Braithwaite complained of a headache one morning, Ms. Stewart immediately took her blood pressure, kindly inquiring about whether her house was too hot ("I get headaches if my house is too hot"). When it turned out that Ms. Braithwaite's blood pressure was high, Ms. Stewart was reassuring ("It's probably just your present circumstances") at the same time that she recommended a Brooklyn doctor. Shortly after, when Ms. Braithwaite was preparing a patient for a bath, Ms. Stewart called out, "I'll come and help you get her out."

Knowing that they would get a sympathetic ear and useful advice, aides came to Ms. Stewart with personal as well as work problems, and on a number of occasions she interceded on their behalf with the nursing administration. Ms. Stewart took it on herself to tutor one Dominican aide in English to help her pass a newly required competency exam, and she successfully encouraged others to continue with their schooling. Aides expressed concern for Ms. Stewart. When she skipped lunch, a common occurrence, aides tried to persuade her to eat and offered to bring a tray up to her.

A woman with enormous pride in her profession, Ms. Stewart tried to instill a similar feeling in the aides. A common refrain was, "This is your house while you are here." Needless to say, aides were not convinced, and they joked with Ms. Stewart when she used the phrase. Yet, interestingly, they did not balk when she criticized them for slipshod work. They respected and liked her, and besides, she made the criticisms in a gentle and kidding way. Unable to fit a box in a nursing-station cabinet, Ms. Roberts simply walked off, leaving the cabinet door open and the shelf's contents askew. Ms. Stewart good-humoredly chided her. "What would you do if this was your kitchen? Think of this as your kitchen." Ms. Roberts backtracked to rearrange the shelf, chatting with Ms. Stewart all the while. When she was through, Ms. Roberts joked, "You got me on that one!" Another time, Ms. Braithwaite went to lunch before getting all her patients up. On return, Ms. Stewart gently rebuked her, and Ms. Braithwaite went off to make amends, without any hard feelings. When aides complained that they had too much work after the shift hours were changed, Ms. Stewart firmly told them they just needed to organize their time better. Aides disagreed, but this did not undercut their warm feelings and admiration for her.

Ms. Stewart consciously worked to develop floor loyalty and raise work morale. To some extent, she succeeded. Certainly, aides liked working on her floor, and two floaters, who had no permanent section, tried to get assigned there. Ms. Stewart's was the only floor to have a weekly floor meeting, which she instituted shortly after she arrived, during which problems and new developments were discussed. At Christmas, Ms. Stewart was the only supervisor to organize gift-giving among her staff, devising a floor raffle whereby aides and nurses bought a present (of no more than $30) for the person whose name they drew. I thought aides would resent this additional burden since many were complaining about the onerous cost of Christmas gifts. I was wrong. Aides were delighted with the arrangement and spent a lot of time thinking about and buying the presents. Ms. Stewart tried hard to be fair in dividing work assignments and benefits. When word came that only three aides on the floor could attend a special social work luncheon in the main dining room, she scrupulously held a drawing to select who would go. Other nursing coordinators arbitrarily assigned aides to attend, and on one floor, the nurse forgot to tell aides altogether.

A nurse like Ms. Stewart can make a difference by creating a congenial work atmosphere and keeping a closer watch on patient care than is the norm. Yet the relationship between nurses' leadership style and aides' job performance is not clear-cut. Despite Ms. Stewart's leadership, one aide on her floor was decidedly lackadaisical in her approach, another extremely competent but gruff with patients. At the other extreme, Ms. Williams was an ineffectual nursing coordinator whose reign is best characterized as one of benign neglect. She largely left the running of the floor to the practical nurse, a bitter woman who lashed out at patients and aides alike and set a tone that certainly would have permitted widespread emotional abuse on the floor. Yet nearly all the aides were extraordinarily conscientious and kind with patients—the best team in the nursing home, according to one social worker. He half-jokingly attributed their closeness to poor leadership, calling them "aides in adversity." The four excellent core aides on this floor had all worked at the Crescent Nursing Home more than fifteen years, much of it together. Deeply committed to doing a good job, they had a strong loyalty to each other and to their patients.[3]

Student Trainees and On-Call Aides

Although nurses are always telling them what to do, aides, at least on the day shift, get some consolation in that they sometimes supervise others, namely, unpaid student trainees and volunteers.

A nearby nursing aide training school sent students, in batches of about ten, to the Crescent Nursing Home for three-week stretches of clinical experience. Trainees were in the home about two-thirds of the year, along with a teacher/supervisor who spent most of the time in the staff dining room. The students were divided equally among the patient floors, usually two to a floor; a nurse on the floor assigned each student to an aide. An aide could count on getting a student trainee for a three-week stint about every three months.

The students were a big help. Aides allocated tasks to them throughout the day: they made beds, dressed and changed patients, fed patients, and helped with baths and lifting. Generally, aides established a maternal relationship with the students, young black and Hispanic women, and rarely were imperious or lost their tempers.

About a dozen high school-aged minority students from a special school for the mentally disabled came to the nursing home daily as part of a work training program. A few of these volunteers were assigned to the nursing department, where their bed-making assistance was especially appreciated by aides. "Thank God Robbie is here now," said one aide who had been worried that the young volunteer who helped her with beds three mornings a week would not show up. "Now I'm great."

While staff aides have no authority to supervise workers in the replacement pool, these on-call aides are in a difficult position. Not guaranteed a full workweek, they never know when their services will be needed, and they are ineligible for benefits that staff aides receive. Frequently, the nursing home asks them to come in at the last minute; most are reluctant to say no, fearing they will be called less often if they refuse. On the job, they must constantly adjust to new routines, new patients, and new co-workers as they move from one floor to another. On-staff aides sometimes assign them unpopular patients at mealtimes and criticize them for making mistakes on the job.

Staff aides, however, have no official power over on-call workers, and, even in the case of student trainees and volunteers, they have nothing like the authority that nurses are allowed over them. Aides are only assigned a student temporarily. Besides, the nursing coordinators and school supervisors decide which tasks the students can do and are the figures to whom the students are ultimately accountable. In truth, aides are at the bottom of the nursing pecking order, and they must suffer the many frustrations that result.

Nurses and Aides: Women's Authority over Women

Nurses and aides alike do "gendered work" in service jobs where women predominate, yet they occupy distinct, unequal, places in the nursing home hierarchy.

For aides, nurses, especially RNs, are the direct agents of bureaucratic control. As aides' immediate supervisors, they enforce and monitor the nursing home's regulations and design work schedules and care plans that dictate how and when aides must look after patients.

That Crescent nurses are women, typically minority women, does not eliminate the effects of their authority. Despite shared gender, aides must follow nurses' orders, even if they disagree. Subtle distinctions, from uniforms to terms of address, emphasize the professional qualifications and superior status of RNs in the institution. Moreover, RNs in particular, concerned with proper procedures and caught up in a web of paperwork, have a less personal, more bureaucratic approach to care than aides, who deal with patients' moment-to-moment needs.

Nurses' leadership style can blunt the impact of their authority and is the key factor in determining how they get along with aides. Nurses face classic dilemmas of middle management, pressed by management demands, from above, and workers' demands, from below. Well-liked nurses are those who make concerted efforts to establish good relations with aides; in doing so, the nurses can draw on racial, ethnic, and gender identities they have in common with aides. At the same time, it is possible that brusque and haughty nurses are resented all the more because aides expect them, as women, often women of color, to be sympathetic and supportive.

Whatever nurses' management style, basic inequalities of status and power between aides and nurses remain. Indeed, all RNs expect and receive a certain amount of deference from aides. I noticed that even the most popular nurses invariably, though perhaps unconsciously, made claims to higher status in conversations with aides by referring to their superior characteristics such as medical knowledge and competence. Most important, all nurses make decisions and issue orders that constrain and limit aides and thus create, for aides, yet another set of caregiving dilemmas.

6

Family Ties

Family relationships—between aides and their families as well as between aides and patients' families—create additional pressures. Feminist scholars have shown that the work place and the family are not two separate spheres but are closely interconnected, two worlds in one, as some call it (Pleck 1976; Zavella 1987). In pointing to ways the home finds its way onto the shop floor, researchers on working-class women provide a broad framework for looking at the situation of nursing aides.

What the literature shows, to begin with, is that many working-class women use family and kinship ties to get their jobs. Often, they gravitate to certain occupations because the hours fit in with their household and child care responsibilities. Many typical female occupations are in fact extensions of women's domestic roles in the family. The world, Arlie Hochschild (1983: 170) writes, turns to women for mothering, and this fact silently attaches itself to many a job description.

By bringing family values and roles to the job, women humanize the work place, to use Louise Lamphere's (1987) phrase. In the factory Lamphere studied, women proudly showed each other family photographs and shared information about their families. Across the Atlantic, in an English factory, sewers "domesticated production" by decorating their machines with pictures of family members and wearing slippers at work (Westwood 1985).

Women's family roles, values, and identities can, in addition, bridge significant divisions at work. Despite racial, ethnic, and other cleavages, women co-workers share experiences as mothers and wives. In a number of settings, "sister" workers are joined together by celebrating rituals that mark life-cycle changes in family roles. Portuguese and Colombian women immigrants in the factory Lamphere (1987) studied, for example, celebrated weddings and baby showers during lunch breaks. In describing the attention and elaborate gifts lavished on pregnant women in an English factory, Sallie Westwood (1985: 228) writes that motherhood was celebrated on the shop floor as the universal and identifying feature of womanhood: "In this, it cut across racial and ethnic divisions, encouraging all women to share in the unity expressed by the mother."

Family ties, feminist scholars also show, have implications for relations with management. Earlier views of women and work—that some women are docile employees because of socialization in the family or, like men, because they fear losing jobs that are important to the family income (Lamphere 1987)—emphasized the ways these ties fostered conservatism. It has been argued, too, that women's commitment to marriage and family may lead to a view of themselves as temporary workers, or a sense that their domestic identities are primary, and a resulting complacency about work conditions (Tentler 1979). And management may co-opt women's family identities, using these identities to build a loyal work force and nonresistant work culture (Lamphere 1985, 1987).

What feminist scholars now emphasize is that family ties can, at times, have the opposite effect. They may form a basis for resistance to management demands. By providing a common set of understandings and values among women workers, family ties can help create a shared—and oppositional—work culture (Benson 1986; Lamphere 1987; Westwood 1985). Karen Sacks (1988) goes further. In her study of Duke Medical Center employees, she argues that the values and organizational and interpersonal skills black women workers learned in the family made it possible for them to stage an effective walkout and begin a union drive.

Much of what feminist scholars have observed in other work settings, we will see, holds true at the Crescent Nursing Home. But there is more. The focus on the pressures nursing aides experience on the job points to additional ways the family impinges on the work place. Although we know a lot about women's difficulties in balancing family and career responsibilities, the emphasis has been on the impact of this juggling act for relations in the home. The question here is how the pressures and obligations of women's family roles influence their experiences and behavior at work.

Furthermore, there is an entirely different aspect to family relations in nursing homes than is found in most other work settings. Unlike a factory or an office, the nursing home as a work place involves the family ties of patients as well. Spouses or children who visit regularly try to continue their caregiving and protective role in the institutional setting, and this creates additional strains and problems for nursing aides.

Nursing Aides' Families

Nursing aides' family ties, values, and relationships enter the nursing home in a number of ways.

FAMILY BONDS AT WORK

Quite a few aides at the Crescent Nursing Home literally bring family members to work. When I was there, on the day shift alone, ten aides had a relative working in the nursing home.[1] One had brought her son in as a porter; another got her brother-in-law a job in the housekeeping department. There were two sister pairs (one, a practical nurse and a nursing aide; the other, two nursing aides) and a mother-daughter combination. There were female in-laws, too: one aide's mother-in-law worked on the evening shift, and one aide's sister-in-law worked in the temporary nursing aide pool. Occasionally, work ties turn into family relationships: two nursing aides met their live-in companions at the Crescent Nursing Home. None of the relatives worked on the same floor, but they often ate and took breaks together and did one another various favors. Indeed, some aides complained among themselves that Ms. Roy had unfairly used influence to place her sister-in-law as a substitute rehabilitation aide for several weeks.

Whether aides are actually related or not, their family roles and identities provide a common ground that brings them together at work. This did not, as in factories studied by some feminist scholars, entail the celebration of life-cycle events. At the Crescent Nursing

Home, there were no baby showers, bridal rituals, or birthday parties. Only rarely did someone bring family pictures to show co-workers. Even then, a woman usually only showed them to her close friends, typically, of the same ethnic group. Nor were the signs of domesticating production that Westwood (1985: 21–22) found among sewers in an English factory present at Crescent. A strict dress code prevailed: wearing slippers—a way, in Westwood's view, of reasserting the domestic presence on the shop floor—was not allowed. And whereas Westwood writes of sewers putting family pictures on their machines, aides at Crescent had no place on the job to put family memorabilia. "Their" rooms were patients' rooms, where patients' family pictures were on display. The only space that was truly theirs, their lockers, was buried deep in the back of the first floor in a dark room. Workers went there as little as possible. (A few Jamaicans spoke of duppies, or spirits of the dead, lurking there.) They kept their lockers padlocked to prevent stealing and only used them to store street clothes and coats.

Despite the lack of life-cycle rituals and family picture displays, the bond the women share as mothers (and to a much lesser extent, as daughters and wives) provides a common set of understandings, worries, and concerns that, at times, bridges ethnic cleavages. As mothers—all but one aide I met had children—aides are the center of a warm and supportive nexus of relationships in the family. They are proud of their children, worry about them, and want them to do well.

To talk about children is to enter friendly territory. A black American and a Haitian worker, who normally had little to do with each other, began a warm and animated conversation about their children's education when they met in the hall. When a Jamaican, a Dominican, and a Guyanese woman sat at lunch talking, inevitably the topic turned to children: to schools, clothes, and whether, in fact, to have more children. A Haitian aide told me how she got accepted among her co-workers when she was new to the floor. "Talk about your family, your kids." I found this true as well. That I was a mother, with a small child, made it easier, I think, for me to be accepted by many workers. Despite the enormous class, educational, and racial differences between us, our shared bond as mothers helped to bridge the gaps. When lunchtime conversations drifted to talk of children, I asked questions and was able to participate in my own role as mother.

A breakthrough in my relations with several workers inadvertently occurred when I happened to have some photographs of my daughter with me. Seeing Lucille Campbell, an aide with whom I had developed a close relationship, I went over to show her the pictures, even though she was eating lunch with two women who had, up to this point, been singularly unfriendly. As the aides passed the pictures around, they viewed me in a new way. For the first time, the two unfriendly workers joked and talked with me good-humoredly. After this, they invariably asked about my daughter when we chatted. Relations warmed with another worker when she learned, one day, that I had to leave early to tend to my sick daughter. As I left the facility, she put her arm around me in a motherly fashion—the first time she had done this—and warmly said that she hoped my daughter would soon feel better. Months after I left the nursing home, when I returned to visit, the first question many workers asked was, "How is your little girl?"

Aides' shared identities, values, and roles as mothers help to underpin a work culture that, as chapter 7 shows, makes the job more bearable and provides a basis for resistance to management, with all the complications this involves in the nursing home context. There is a conservative side to family ties as well. Workers are generally reluctant to push their opposition to management policies into direct confrontations, unless they have clear-cut union backing and protection, for fear of endangering the jobs that are so crucial to their family's economic well-being. They swallow unpleasant orders because, as one woman put it, "We have no other choice but to do what we gotta do."

It is important to emphasize, however, that family roles do not make aides complacent or "collusive" with management. Aides have a keen sense of their opposition to management, and they share interests and commitments with each other as workers. In describing why aides on her floor, who were of varied ethnic groups, got along so well, Ms. Watson summed up two key and related identities of Crescent nursing aides: "We are mothers, and we are workers."

Nor do family roles lead aides to see themselves as temporary workers. Although some said they wished they could quit work altogether or work part-time, they knew this was not realistic. All were committed, for the money and the benefits, to full-time work for a full-length working career. Indeed, those in the temporary pool were longing to become full-time workers. Giving birth did not interfere with women's work careers at the Crescent Nursing Home. Those who had children while on staff took all, or part, of the ten months unpaid maternity leave allowed and then returned to work.

CARING WORK

The nursing aide job itself draws heavily on women's roles as mothers—something, of course, that sharply differentiates it from industrial labor. Indeed, aides, as well as others, view the job as an extension of their nurturant family roles. The physical aspects of the job involve "mothering work," for example, giving baths, making beds, feeding patients, and fixing patients' hair. And there is emotional caring as well.

Hochschild (1983: 7) has coined the phrase "emotional labor" to describe labor requiring workers, in their contact with the public, to induce or suppress feelings—to create a "publicly observable facial and bodily display"—in order to produce the proper state of mind in others. Flight attendants, for example, the focus of her study, must smile and show warmth to passengers whatever their actual feelings. Hochschild (ibid., 181) notes that because women are schooled in emotion management at home, they have entered, in disproportionate numbers, those jobs calling for emotional labor outside the home.

Nursing aides doubtless do put on a false face much of the day as they manage emotions in caring for patients. But, unlike flight attendants, who have fleeting contacts with passengers, nursing aides care for the same few patients day after day. Many become genuinely emotionally attached to patients. While Hochschild (ibid., 187) suggests that "emotional laborers" who sincerely offer warm, personal service do so on behalf of the company, this is not the case at the Crescent Nursing Home. Sincerely compassionate and kind aides at Crescent are, in a sense, their own agents, expressing their own feelings for patients and their own views of how to behave. Indeed, as we saw in chapter 4, aides are sometimes warm and supportive in spite of and in direct opposition to the nursing home administration and supervisors. What is significant here is that in providing emotional comfort and nurturance to patients, whether feigned or from the heart, aides are applying skills and patterns of behavior they have learned and practiced in their unpaid caregiving roles at home.

For many, the opportunity to do "caring work" outside the home is an enormous source of satisfaction. Many aides spoke of the rewards they received from "doing good for people" and having patients need them. "They depend on you," said Florence Wright. "You get a satisfaction from seeing you've cleaned them and met a lot of their wants. Sometimes they need someone to listen to them."

Some aides likened relationships with patients to those they had in their own families. Ms. Darius compared taking care of patients with nursing her husband when he was sick. A few said that patients filled in, in some ways, for their own absent or dead parents or grandparents. One worker said, "I never had a grandmother or grandfather; here I find them." An aide who grew up in Georgia and came to New York in the 1960s, explained, "You grow to love the patients. It's like a family to me 'cause I don't have no family in New York."

Most common, there was the comparison of patients with children. In describing their job, many aides explicitly used the child care analogy. "If you've ever been a mother," said one devoted aide, "it's like taking care of children." Or as another put it, more bluntly, in trying to capture the difficulties of her job, "You ever have to look after ten babies?"

Such characterizations do not necessarily indicate negative attitudes and poor care. Nursing staff have come under attack in the literature for their tendency to think of and treat patients like children. The criticism is that such infantilization is patronizing, humiliating, and authoritarian; undermines residents' sense of dignity and self-worth; leads to not taking patients seriously; predisposes staff to respond in predetermined ways; and actually encourages, in the manner of a self-fulfilling prophecy, regressive behavior among residents (Shield 1988; Kayser-Jones 1990).

To be sure, infantilizing treatment frequently does have these negative effects. Yet a maternal stance often reflects genuine affection (Retsinas, quoted in Shield 1988: 198). It may also, as Lore Wright (1988) suggests, get results, as when confused residents respond to baby talk rather than normal terms of address.[2] What I found, moreover, was that verbal characterizations and actual treatment did not always correspond. Many aides who described their jobs to me as akin to taking care of children actually treated patients with respect and did not infantilize them. This includes the saintlike Ana, portrayed in chapter 4, who was one of the most sympathetic and caring aides in the nursing home. Given residents' overwhelming dependence on aides for help with the most basic tasks of daily living, aides' verbal characterizations of patients as childlike are not irrational (Retsinas, quoted in Shield 1988: 198).

If caregiving is, in some respects, like mothering away from home, there is another way that aides' role as mothers enters the facility. A few aides had developed special links with alert female residents, based in part on their shared role as mothers. These elderly women sympathized with and occasionally advised younger aides on child-rearing and childbearing matters. Sometimes, they complained together about relations with men. And, finally, it is worth noting that while I was there, two aides—among the "saints" I spoke of earlier—brought their own children to the nursing home to meet patients they had spoken so much about at home.

FAMILY PRESSURES AT WORK

Nursing aides' family responsibilities add to the seemingly endless strains they experience on the job. It is not just that they must perform the caregiving role, with its attendant emotional and physical demands, around the clock (on the second shift in the home as well as in the work place). The pressures of family roles and obligations do not disappear when they enter the work place. They are a common source of strain that can, at times, affect caring for "strangers" at work.

This is not to characterize aides' family lives, as one recent study does, in such unrelentingly adverse terms as "unkind," "oppressive," and "leaving deep scars on emotional life" or to describe most aides as "living precariously on the edge" (Tellis-Nayak and Tellis-Nayak 1989). Like other scholars of black American and Caribbean immigrant family life, I found that nursing aides were deeply involved with and received enormous satisfaction from their children; many had developed close, working relationships with their spouses; and most were enmeshed in a large, supportive network of kin.

The women I met were struggling financially to make a decent life for themselves and their children, usually with help from others in their household. Married or not, most aides had steady live-in partners who worked. Older aides sometimes got help from adult children who lived with them, and a number of women, who owned their homes, rented out rooms or apartments. Consider three women I have mentioned many times. Ms. Roy's husband worked as a factory supervisor; Nina Acosta lived in a rent-free apartment thanks to her husband's job as the building's superintendent. Older, and more established, Ms. Riley rented out an apartment in her house; the man she lived with worked as a cab driver; and a grown son, a mechanic, who also lived with her, helped out as well. Half of the fourteen women for whom I have detailed financial information had annual household incomes over $45,000; another three, between $30,000 and $40,000. The four in the bottom category, between $20,000 and $25,000, had to get by with no other financial help.

Whether or not aides had a steady live-in partner, they bore the burden of the "second shift," like most American women (Hochschild 1989). In addition to the physical and emotional demands of work, they had to manage household chores and, in the case of mothers of young children (and a few grandmothers who cared for small grandchildren), complicated baby-sitting arrangements that wore them down.[3]

Many husbands did help out, for example, with shopping, the laundry, taking children to school, and occasionally cooking. As children got older, they also took on household responsibilities. Still, the lion's share fell on aides. "I'm always working," is how Ms. Darius, a Haitian woman with eight children, put it. Although her husband, a mechanic, does not help much around the house ("Some men are like that"), her mother, who lives with her, certainly does. Nonetheless, there is a lot to do. "I have to work twenty-four hours. When I go home, I take a nap, then get up again; sometimes I get up at two in the morning, iron for the children and go back to sleep" (cf. Pessar 1987, on Dominican garment workers in New York).

Day shift aides with young children have to arrange early-morning child care so they can leave home sometime between 5:00 A.M. and 6:00 A.M. to be at work by 7:00. Those few with a live-in mother are the luckiest. Some, like Ms. Tate, rely on husbands to get the children ready. A Jamaican woman with three daughters, ranging in age from five to fourteen, Ms. Tate has a long trip to work from her central Brooklyn home, involving a bus and subway ride. She leaves home at 5:45 every morning, before her children are awake. The eldest two get ready and go to school on their own; they have keys to let themselves in the house after school. Her husband takes the youngest to school in the morning; Ms. Tate picks her daughter up from an after-school program on the way home from work, after which she settles into her household routine of cooking, doing laundry, and making the children's lunches.

Others, like Ms. Roy, wake their children very early to get them to a baby-sitter before setting off to work. She takes her two children to a woman who lives a few blocks away before getting into the subway at about 6:00 A.M. The baby-sitter cares for the little girl all day long (along with her own children); she puts the six-year-old boy on the school bus in the morning and waits for him to get off in the afternoon. Ms. Roy is pleased with the current baby-sitter. The previous one, it turned out, had distributed Ms. Roy's son's antibiotics to all the children in her care so that the boy was constantly ill with infections. On top of the typical childhood accidents and illnesses that periodically crop up, several aides have to cope with additional worries: children with special health problems requiring hospitalization or regular doctor visits—asthma and neurological disorders, to mention two cases.

For nearly all, given their neighborhoods and local schools, there is concern about their children's safety as well as educational progress. Worried about drugs in school, Maria Castillo was trying to arrange a transfer for her daughter. Those who can manage the fees—and a substantial number make enormous financial sacrifices to do so—send their children to Catholic schools.[4] Many aides spoke of how they strictly supervised after-school play, not allowing children out on the street because they feared crime and mixing with the wrong crowd. All were concerned that their children do well in school and not end up in jobs like their own. (Many older aides' children, in fact, had attained white-collar or highly skilled manual positions.)

Added to the burdens of work and home routines, a significant number also fit various educational courses into their demanding and exhausting schedules. Of the fourteen day shift aides I formally interviewed, ten had taken one or more courses at some point in their careers, usually in their twenties, thirties, and forties, when they were young enough to realistically contemplate a career change. Several had gone to classes to prepare for the high school equivalency examination; a few had taken classes in such areas as key punch operation and word processing (though because of the better salaries and benefits, they stayed in their jobs at the Crescent Nursing Home); many had gone to the free nursing aide training courses offered by the union to become certified or to update their certification; and two were currently attending night classes to qualify to become LPNs. Ms. Etienne, a thirty-year-old Haitian woman with four children, was one of these. For two years she went to college, three evenings a week, for LPN training. She officially became an LPN at Crescent shortly after I left, and she was already arranging to go on for an RN qualification. She managed because her husband, a limousine driver, looked after the children while she was at school and when she had to study.

How do these family demands and concerns impinge on aides'

work lives? They can, for one thing, influence the shift they decide to work. When hired, women indicate their shift preference, and later they can request a change. While aides disagree over which shift is better for raising children and running a family, some had specifically chosen their shift, and in a few cases had to forgo their preference, to combine work with household responsibilities.

Several aides, for example, preferred the evening or night shift but had to work days for family reasons. "When I was 3–11," Ms. Etienne told me, "I didn't have time to see my family. When I came home, they [the children] were sleeping, and when I left they weren't there." Also, her husband did not like having to put the children to bed. Ana had been happy on the night shift, but she frequently had to leave her twelve-year-old daughter home alone when she went to work. "She was lonely, she couldn't sleep. She tell me she was scared of sleeping alone. I was worried about her so I changed with someone."

Typically, the effect of family pressures is to add to the burdens of aides' emotional labor: they take a toll on the workers rather than the patients. The average, basically kindhearted and decent aide does not take out her everyday family woes or anxieties on patients or sink into apathy or indifference. As in other kinds of emotion work, most aides, most of the time, mask their own personal worries under cover of a kindly veneer. This is a basic part of the job, business as usual. Indeed, caring for and becoming involved with patients sometimes takes their minds off their own concerns.

No matter how tired or worried about personal troubles, the truly excellent aides continue to be nurturant and supportive. One day Ana was under enormous strain. Not only did she have a terrible migraine headache but she was also distressed because her apartment had been partially destroyed by a fire the night before. It took an enormous effort, but she was warm, comforting, and diligent in her work the entire day. The same was true of Ms. Roy, who worried constantly that her son, who was subject to seizures, would have one when she was at work ("When a call comes for me, my heart is in my mouth, imagining the worst"). Both Ms. Roy and Ana talked to their alert patients about their own troubles. More commonly, when aides have special problems, they chat with co-workers as they work and at breaks.

There are some times, however, when the aides' family pressures do have negative effects for patients. Aides are occasionally so exhausted by the combination of work, home, and, sometimes, school demands that they simply drag themselves around at work in an apathetic way.

With most aides, this is a rare occurrence and usually only happens when there are special crises at home. Moreover, once in a while, a few "do a double" for the extra money—work a double shift or sixteen hours straight—and toward the end of their work hours, they have little energy left. For a handful, a kind of listlessness with patients is a more or less permanent state, and I think, as in the case of one aide training to be a practical nurse, their overtired condition is at least partly responsible.

Family emergencies or crises, for example, a sick child at home or a husband's illness, are, understandably, often distracting. Ms. Tate was upset one day because her daughter was ill. Her mind was far from her patients, and she did her job in a mechanical, unfeeling way. Unable to telephone from the floor, she constantly tried to get downstairs to use the pay telephone to see how her daughter was. I even saw her trying to call from a patient's private telephone, something, if discovered or reported, that could have meant her job. Aides cannot receive personal telephone calls on their floor, but emergency calls, which are sometimes put through, can upset aides and affect patient care. One afternoon, Ms. Renald was called to the telephone: it was a doctor investigating possible child abuse by asking about a bad burn her daughter had suffered. Deeply disturbed by the accusation, Ms. Renald told me how her daughter had been accidentally burned in the bath. She could not focus well on her work and was offhand with patients the rest of the day.

Patients' Families

Nursing aides have to contend with patients' families as well as their own, which often brings added headaches. "Their family makes things worse for us," said one aide, and most others would heartily agree.

PATIENT FAMILY INVOLVEMENT

Patients' family members are an ongoing part of the nursing home scene. Most American families, studies show, do not "dump" their relatives in nursing homes and ignore them (Johnson and Grant 1985). Many family members try to continue their caregiving role after their spouse or parent is institutionalized, and visiting by family members is common. Not surprisingly, research documents that this contact has positive effects for residents' psychosocial well-being (Greene and Monahan 1982) and can even improve the quality of family relationships (Smith and Bengtson 1979).

On the basis of her participant observation study in a New England nursing home, Shield (1988: 59–60) sums up the positive role of actively involved family members: they are arbiters, promulgators, and nurturers. They provide such valuable services as doing errands and ensuring that clothing is properly mended and cleaned. By interceding on residents' behalf and talking to social workers or administrators about specific matters, such as overheated rooms, they can protect their relatives (see also Savishinsky 1991). And they soften institutional existence by bringing homemade or special foods residents prefer.

Family members often perform these roles at the Crescent Nursing Home. Although many come once a week or less, a sizable number are regulars, coming almost every day, some for a few hours and some for even longer. During my research, there were about twenty regular family visitors on the day shift and about the same number in the early evening. In fact, many families had sought out the Crescent Nursing Home precisely because it was near their homes and they could visit often. Although most regulars lived in the neighborhood, a few traveled long distances every day (in several cases, more than an hour and a half each way) to see their parent or spouse.

The regulars not only provide residents with companionship and support—soothing and reassuring the anxious, depressed, and confused—but also watch over them and monitor care. And they perform some basic bed and body work. Many fed their spouses or parents lunch or dinner. Often, they helped residents get dressed and cleaned up after them. Some brought residents downstairs to the main dining room and, on nice days, to the rooftop deck. They organized clothes and occasionally did all the laundry. And there were lots of little chores or comforts they provided, like pouring a glass of water when their relative was thirsty or fetching items for the bedridden.

AIDES' REACTIONS

What is the nursing aides' reaction to such family involvement? One might expect them to be pleased when patients' relatives visit frequently and assume some of their work burden such as serving meals and sorting laundry. Quantitative studies, using checklists to gather ratings from nursing staff and family concerning who should do various tasks, also point in this direction. For the most part, relatives and staff agree on who should do what (Rubin and Shuttlesworth 1983; Schwartz and Vogel 1990).

Yet far from being grateful to family visitors, I found that nursing aides tended to be annoyed, occasionally deeply angry, with them. The general view is that actively involved relatives are another source of pressure on the job.

It is not that family members are thought to be infringing on tasks that aides claim as their own. Indeed, aides generally take for granted assistance that family members offer. Aides have come to expect that certain regulars will do specific jobs, like helping with meals, and they build such assistance into their own schedules. When these relatives do not show up, aides are irritated since now their routines are upset and they have what they perceive to be added work. Take the case of Mr. Rubin. Despite his own serious health problems, including a bad back and a heart condition, he came every day to feed lunch to his wife, a woman suffering from the late stages of Alzheimer's disease. On some days, she seemed unable to recognize him, though generally he had a calming effect on her. When Mr. Rubin fed his wife, she ate much better than when aides tried to do it; he sat next to her, in the hall, coaxing her slowly and patiently to eat spoonful by spoonful. Occasionally, when he did not turn up, the aides' normal routine was disrupted in that they had one more, very difficult, person to feed. They understood that Mr. Rubin was probably ill, but they were annoyed nonetheless.

Aides do in fact feel sorry for many relatives, like Mr. Rubin, who wear themselves out, physically and emotionally, by their daily visits. Moreover, some aides get along well with family members and go out of their way to keep them up to date about the patients' condition and to try to cheer them up despite the unhappy circumstances. As with patients, what aides appreciate about family members is not material gifts or presents, which a few gave, but personal concern for them as people. Vanessa Clifton was clearly pleased that a number of residents' relatives sent her cards and letters when she was out sick for several months. What gratified Ms. Price was not that a resident's husband spent money on a book to help her study for the high school equivalency exam—he, too, spent his time by his wife's side studying for the exam—but that he sincerely wanted to assist her.

This said, however, the common view among aides is that patients' relatives interfere and make life more difficult for them.[5] This view is summed up well in a conversation I had with Ms. Price, an aide with four patients in her section who had family visitors who came virtually every day. When I once commented at lunch on the number of family visitors in her section, she assumed I was sympathizing with her and said, with enormous appreciation, "Thank you. You see the problems I have." Ever-present relatives, in short, spell trouble, and an aide with many in her section is considered unlucky. A couple of aides even mentioned patients' families as the biggest problem they had in doing their job.

A major reason for this is that patients' relatives are thought to be too demanding. "They feel," said one worker, "you never doing enough." Or as another put it, "Some of them don't want the mother home, but when they come to the nursing home, they want her perfect. But when you have ten patients, you cannot give them that kind of care." A common complaint about regular family visitors is that they think their relative is the only patient. "I can't stand that woman," said Ms. James, referring to a resident's daughter. "She comes round saying, you have to reposition my mother NOW. I was busy with someone else."

Relatives may insist on a level of care that the aide would not normally provide. One resident's sister, who came every day, made an issue of the need to put her relative in pants instead of a dress, which other female residents wore. This made more work for the aide, who explained that putting pants on the resident was extremely difficult, much more difficult than a dress.

In general, relatives who are around make requests that residents themselves are not able or do not bother to express. Concerned with their relatives' welfare and often physically unable to cope with problems that arise, family members have a sense of urgency that aides do not share. A wet bed, a resident who has slipped down in a chair, food that has spilled on the floor—these, to aides, are the realities of nursing home life. If an aide is in the midst of bathing or cleaning a patient, she will not want to interrupt this procedure—which, after all, often means leaving the patient naked or in an uncomfortable position—to deal with what she regards as a minor and routine matter. When relatives ask her to see to their relatives and abandon the task at hand, aides are irritated. That they must, moreover, suppress this annoyance and be polite adds to their difficulties.

Jean Hunt, viewed as an especially demanding relative, constantly put her mother's aide in this position. In her late sixties and in poor health herself, she came every day, rain or shine, to see her ninety-eight-year-old mother. Ms. Price, the aide, sympathized with Jean's problems—having to deal with her deep attachment to her mother, who was bound to die soon, and her own ailing health. Never once did I see Ms. Price express irritation or anger toward Jean. Ms. Price was always calm and polite, even when she was the object of Jean's outbursts. To me, however, Ms. Price complained about what a trial Jean was. There seemed to be an endless stream of requests—to clean up, remake the bed, change her mother—when Ms. Price was in the midst of tending to other patients. If Ms. Price did not respond immediately, Jean was visibly piqued and, later, often exploded.

If relatives are annoyed, there is always the possibility that they will take their complaints and demands to higher authorities, a distinct drawback from the aides' point of view. They may complain to social services and other higher-ups; at the least, they might cause a nursing administrator or social worker to ask questions.

Family complaints and demands may be all the more irritating and carry added symbolic weight because they come from people of higher class and racial status. Most family visitors at Crescent are middle class and white; virtually all aides, working-class women of color. Social class and racial differences often reinforce, in subtle and unconscious ways, the relatives' sense that aides are there to serve them. For the aides' part, they may be especially sensitive to signs of condescension and superior attitudes and behavior from white, better-off relatives.

Whether regular visitors complain or not, aides feel that they spoil patients by lavishing attention on them and raising expectations of care. This is true of undemanding relatives as well as those with constant complaints. Take Mr. Rubin once again. In many ways, he was the ideal relative. Careful to cultivate good relations with his wife's aide, he hardly ever complained or asked for anything. He sat quietly with his wife, helping out with many tasks and even assisting other patients in her room. Much as aides liked him personally and sympathized with his situation, they saw him as causing problems: his constant presence spoiled his wife. By giving her the kind of attention they were unable to provide, he got her used to a relatively high level of care. When he left, she was, they felt, more difficult than before, whining and crying and inconsolable. And if he did not show up at all, she was especially hard to manage.

Of less importance but still a factor is that family members sometimes create problems for aides by interfering with care. In these cases, relatives are intruding on technical aspects of care that aides—and nurses—think are beyond relatives' purview. The general principle of task allotment is not an issue. As noted, aides readily accept relatives' help in such "technical" or instrumental tasks as feeding patients, making beds, and cleaning that are officially aides' duties. Aides view relatives' help as interference when it adds to their work load or contradicts the nurse's orders, possibly harming patients and getting the aides into trouble.

Jean Hunt, the demanding daughter, is a perfect example. Upset that her mother was physically restrained in bed, Jean often removed the restraints even though she was repeatedly told by the nurse in charge why they had to be in place. As a result, one afternoon, the old woman fell out of bed, onto the floor. Luckily, she was not hurt, but obviously this was dangerous. What the aide focused on was having to lift the resident to put her back in bed: more, heavy, work.

On a different floor, nurses and aides suspected another demanding regular, Mrs. Adams, of causing her husband, a heavy, paralyzed man suffering from severe dementia, to slide down in his chair by trying, ineffectively and improperly, to reposition him and make him more comfortable. Aides, once more, had to lift and move him to sit him up straight. This was an enormous strain since Mr. Adams was so heavy and could not help. Nurses and aides also believed that Mrs. Adams imagined symptoms, like pains and headaches, that were not there; she demanded medication and immediate treatment that nursing staff were not allowed to give without a doctor's permission.

RELATIVES' GRIEVANCES

Family members, of course, have a long list of their own grievances. In interviews with family members in a Wisconsin nursing home, Bowers (1990) found them to be deeply upset by the staff's failure to provide protective, as opposed to purely technical, care. They were distressed when their relatives were treated in a demeaning or insulting way—made to feel like nuisances, difficult to care for, or that they had unreasonable requests—and when their relatives' emotional needs, personal preferences, and unique personal histories were ignored or overlooked.

These are issues, too, for regular family visitors I met at the Crescent Nursing Home. What figured even more prominently in their complaints, however, at least in conversations with me and at family council meetings, is aides' failure to provide competent technical care and their lack of responsiveness to relatives' own requests and difficulties.

Over and over, family members pointed to failings in care: the husband who wore no special stockings when his wife arrived, though these had been ordered by the doctor; the ulcers on one man's grandmother as well as roommates who were not being fed; and the husband whose eating patterns were not checked properly, though he had serious eating difficulties, which once, before he came to Crescent, required him to be hospitalized for dehydration. Typically, family members blamed aides, the direct agents of care, for the problems. Lost laundry was a universal problem that most were resigned to. As one grandson said, "I take it as a factor of life that you lose all your clothing here."

Family members complained, too, about aides' unsympathetic attitudes to them and unhelpful, sometimes antagonistic, behavior. Family members are often overwhelmed, sometimes to the point of tears, by the helplessness entailed in asking staff busy with other priorities to attend to a relative's needs—something that drives home the fact that their relative's care is no longer in their hands. Often, they are humiliated and upset by having to plead with or cajole aides to get them to meet requests (Hooyman and Lustbader 1986: 302). Understandably, family members are distressed when aides are not responsive, ignore requests, or show signs of hostility.

Mrs. Bernard was especially vocal in her criticisms at one family council meeting I attended. Her characterization of aides was blunt: "When you ask them something, they never answer." She went on, "A patient in my husband's room threw a tray with food all over the room and over my husband's bed. So I didn't want to leave it like that. I asked for a broom, and the aide tells me where to get it. I have a bad back, she didn't even offer to help. In my opinion they're underworked and overpaid." That Mrs. Bernard was expressing the anger and frustrations of many other family members was clear in that other relatives at the meeting all nodded in agreement.

Like others, Mrs. Bernard was annoyed that her requests and instructions were often disregarded. "I left a laundry bag to put dirty laundry in every day," she told the crowd at the meeting. "I explained it to the aides and left a big sign. What do you think? I come and the laundry is not in the bag." Around the room, the family members were abuzz with comments like, "She's bringing up all our points," and "It's true." A frail old woman chimed in, "I come every night to feed my mother who is visually impaired and they expect me to put a bib on her, to prop her up, and I really cannot do this. It is very hard for me."

Perhaps one of the most interesting cases is Mrs. Adams, one of the "demanding regulars" already mentioned. She wrestled with the political dilemma of criticizing black workers whose causes she and her husband championed. Mr. Adams had been a well-known figure on the political Left, to which both he and his wife devoted their lives and for which they made many sacrifices. She was deeply upset over the inadequate care she felt her husband received, and she had nothing but criticism for his nursing aide. Her feeling was that aides, as union members, should be better workers than nonunion employees.

Ill herself (she suffered from a stroke a few years before), it was more than she could bear to come day after day and see instructions ignored or her husband left in an unhealthy state. Having bought undershirts to keep him warm, she arrived to find that his room was cold and he had no undershirt on. Despite the doctor's recommendations, aides continued to use small incontinence briefs that gave her husband a rash or, alternatively, left him in open briefs, which resulted in a wet bed. She thought he was uncomfortable in his chair and not positioned properly and even suspected that a cut he got one evening, which needed stitches, was a result of negligent care in the shower. On top of all this, when she made any comment, the aide, a feisty West Indian and, indeed, one of the worst aides in the nursing home, often snapped at her.

At a family council meeting she summed up her frustrations. "If the nursing aide is not functioning properly, they come to me and say he's a problem. I say I know he's a problem. I was looking after him at home for years, I couldn't do it anymore. That's why he's here. They're union workers, paid union wages, and if they don't work, they should go." In response, all the relatives in the room enthusiastically clapped and cheered.

Usually, relatives keep such complaints to themselves, and it is only in private conversations, well out of the earshot of staff, that they express their views. Even at family council meetings, most relatives are diplomatic in the way they couch their dissatisfactions. Many were only spurred on to air their views at one meeting by the angry comments of Mrs. Bernard and Mrs. Adams, who were seen as bold to be so honest and vocal. Even Mrs. Adams told me, "Of course, I wouldn't say anything to the aide." Family members do not want to antagonize aides, which might result in worse treatment for relatives and more uncomfortable visits for themselves. Some fear that if they complain directly to the aide, or if word gets back of complaints to higher-ups, their relatives will suffer retaliation. Others come to have a sense of hopelessness: whatever they do, nothing will change anyway.

To say that relatives have complaints does not, of course, necessarily mean that their relationships with aides are continually conflict-ridden or even seriously strained. Typically, regulars develop a tolerable working relationship with their relative's aides. Just as there are sources of irritation on both sides which develop day after day, so, too, there are times when they chat about the patient and even work together to help him or her. Usually, they become accustomed to each other, and a level of cordiality is maintained. Often, their relationship extends to asking about each other's health and family. Many family members had, in fact, become attached to their relative's aides and were seriously troubled when the administration proposed to rotate aides.

Relatives who have extremely hostile relations with an aide are unusual. In fact, when tensions become too serious, the social service department generally intervenes, sometimes because the aide herself has complained of insults or difficult relations. In such cases, social workers talk with family members about the problem, with the hope of making them sensitive to aides' feelings. As a last resort, arrangements are made to switch aides so that relatives can start out on a new footing.

Conclusion

Family ties, clearly, are closely interwoven with work in the nursing home context. Aides cannot escape from patients' families, no matter how much they might want to do so, and their own family relationships and responsibilities impinge on their work lives in innumerable ways, often adding to the stresses of the job.

The term "nursing home" suggests a familylike environment. Though, as many point out, the term is a misnomer—Bruce Vladeck

(1980) aptly entitles a chapter in his book, *Unloving Care*, "No Place Like Home"—nursing aides are, in effect, family substitutes, expected to fill caregiving functions associated with the family in an institutional setting. In fact, aides' work draws and builds on and simultaneously reinforces their role and identity as nurturant caregivers in their own families. Aides, however, are more than mother figures in a work context. On the job, they develop a strong sense of their identity as workers, and their relations with each other are significant for their own, as well as patients', lives. Ties with co-workers are a source of comfort and help for aides, but they can also create additional demands and pressures. This is the subject of the next chapter.

7

Work Culture in the Nursing Home

What happens when informal work cultures develop in the nursing home? It is one thing when workers create a culture of their own, with unofficial rules, customs, and understandings, on the factory floor; it is quite another when the setting is a nursing home where patients, not inanimate objects, are the "products and objects" of work (Goffman 1961).

What kind of work culture have aides shaped at the Crescent Nursing Home? In what ways does the work culture—and co-worker relations generally—help aides cope with their jobs but at the same time pose still another set of caregiving dilemmas? And how does the work culture affect patients in the institution?

What has been written about work cultures, mainly in industrial settings, provides important guides for this analysis. Yet, the special nature of the nursing home and paid caregiving adds new dimensions to aides' work culture and gives rise to distinct problems for them.

Work Cultures

By now, we have a large number of studies, mostly of the factory floor, showing how workers create informal work cultures apart from the employer's official regulations. Whether in a garment factory or a chemical plant, work cultures benefit employees in many ways, ranging from reducing job dissatisfaction to fostering worker solidarity and enabling workers to exert some control over production and their work situation. Indeed, Susan Benson and Barbara Melosh's frequently cited definition of work culture—"the ideology and practice with which workers stake out a relatively autonomous sphere of action on the job"—emphasizes how employees distance themselves from the impact of formal authority structures as they confront the limitations and exploit the possibilities of their jobs (Benson 1986: 228).

Informal work cultures have what a number of writers call a dual character, involving both adaptation and resistance (see Benson 1986; Costello 1988; di Leonardo 1985; Lamphere 1985, 1987; Kanter and Stein 1979). For one, there are various coping strategies. Workers in low-skilled and repetitious jobs invent games and rituals and forge relationships and involvements, outside of the official set of tasks and assignments, that create a bit of excitement and drama out of otherwise drab routines (Kanter and Stein 1979).

Among women, we read about wedding rituals and showers celebrated at work (Lamphere 1987; Sacks 1988; Westwood 1985); among male factory workers, about gambling and cardplaying in free time (e.g., Halle 1984). In a wonderful account of "banana time" in a Chicago factory, Donald Roy (1958) shows how a combination of horseplay, conversation, and frequent sharing of food and drink kept machine operators from "going nuts" in their monotonous jobs. Every morning, one worker would snatch and gulp down a coworker's banana, calling out "banana time"; later in the day, rituals of peach time, window time, fish time, and the coke game followed. In the same factory, many years later, "making out," a series of games in which operators tried to achieve production levels that could earn incentive pay, made time pass more quickly and gave workers a sense of pride and accomplishment (Burawoy 1979).

By making work more bearable, these informal activities can serve the ends of the company. Some contend they are a kind of safety valve, channeling dissatisfactions into practices that, in the long run, play a role in workers' adaptation to oppressive conditions and accommodation to employers' demands. In Michael Burawoy's (1979) phrase, work cultures can help to "manufacture consent" to management rules and even motivate workers to push themselves to work hard to advance the interests of the organization.

In contrast, informal work cultures can generate resistance to managerial prerogatives and control. This is the aspect of work cultures that has, of late, been of particular interest to scholars focusing on women's work (Benson 1986; Cooper 1987; Costello 1988; Lamphere 1987; Morgen 1990; Paules 1991; Shapiro-Perl 1984; Sacks 1988; Westwood 1985). A key issue in the literature concerns the conditions that make women's work culture an effective basis for resistance to management. Recent studies of women factory workers and even a few studies of service employees eagerly search for aspects of work culture that are oppositional in character—that give women in low-status, poorly paid, and tedious jobs some control over oppressive conditions, provide a basis for collective action to challenge these working conditions, and afford women ways to advance their interests on the job.

In some ways, the work culture among nursing home aides operates as industrial work studies describe, but in other ways, it is unique. Opposition to management, as well as everyday coping strategies, take on new complexities in personal caring jobs, where, in addition to workers and management, a third, critical, group is involved: people the workers are hired to serve and care for.

In the nursing home, our sympathy, as outside observers, for the workers' plight is complicated by our concern for the frail, sick elderly who are the workers' charges. Inevitably, patients are affected by the work culture that develops, sometimes for the better and sometimes for the worse. What stands out, especially given our focus on the demands on aides, is that elements of resistance embodied in women's work culture can, in the nursing home context, exert pressure on workers to stint on care or ignore abuses of co-workers and thus harm patients that conscientious workers would prefer to protect.

Other pressures from co-workers also impinge on nursing aides. Interpersonal conflicts among them, often intensified by ethnic divisions, can create additional strains.

Making Life at the Bottom Bearable

First, there are the "adaptive" aspects of nursing aides' work culture—for workers and, often, for patients, too. A number of informal social practices and customs have developed among aides that liven up the day and ease the work burden, making a "life at the bottom," as Rosabeth Moss Kanter and Barry Stein (1979) characterize it. On occasion, these practices create problems for patients. Yet to the extent that the aides' informal practices and customs make them happier and help them to adjust to difficult working conditions, then the nursing home organization and, most important, patients frequently benefit. Informal patterns of help among workers can also result in better physical, as well as emotional, care.

The work culture among Crescent aides has its roots in their common occupation, class, gender, race, and immigrant status. Obviously, their shared work interests and problems are critical. Common concerns as mothers and wives also underpin and give a particular tone to the work culture. That all are working class is another important bond. And all share the special burdens and problems that come with minority status and, for the overwhelming majority, being immigrants from the Caribbean region.

Granted, nursing aide work is not as tedious as most factory jobs, where workers spend long days doing simple repetitive work. Although aides take care of the same patients, day after day, and do basically the same routine chores, patients are not machines. Unless residents are comatose, they respond, react, and talk; crises invariably occur on the floor that, no matter how unpleasant, vary the routine. Yet in the nursing home, as on the shop floor, the work culture that has developed knits aides together and adds an important dimension of sociability and interest to the job.

SOCIALIZING AND SELLING

On the patient floors, workers joke, talk, and chat with each other whenever they get the chance. Often, this means a brief encounter when passing in the hall. Although officially against the rules, some manage to cluster in groups of two or three in patient rooms for conversations for a few minutes at various times of the day.

Administrators argue that this kind of informal socializing interferes with care: instead of talking with each other, aides should spend more time looking after and talking with patients. On the whole, however, short conversations among aides on the floor have few negative effects. Often, they put aides in a better mood for dealing with residents. On many occasions, workers vented their irritation at patients in conversation with each other rather than getting angry at patients themselves. I did not get the sense, as Gubrium (1975) did in his study, that aides rushed through their bed and body work to spend time chatting with each other. In fact, on the day shift, most had hardly any time when they were not busy with work tasks. They rarely spent more than ten or fifteen minutes a day, if that much, talking with co-workers when they were not also involved in some kind of patient care. Only a few negligent aides let informal socializing take priority over patient care.

Women from the same ethnic group tend to gravitate to each other, but given the ethnic diversity of the floor work force, this is not always possible. On each patient floor, aides from different ethnic backgrounds can be seen huddling together in conversation or chatting in the hall. Mealtime, in the dayroom, is another opportunity for interaction. Even aides who are most attentive to residents often carry on lively conversations with each other as they feed and encourage residents to eat. As usual, talk centers on such topics as family matters, including children, work complaints, vacations, their own health woes, or sensational events in the news.

It would be a mistake, of course, to ignore some of the problems of the aides' informal social life. On the factory floor, informal conversations and joking and clowning, at worst, slow down production. In "people work," those being served can suffer, especially in total institutions like nursing homes where patients are so dependent on staff (Goffman 1961). (Clientele in restaurants and stores may suffer, too, when waitresses or clerks chat with each other instead of serving them or make rude remarks within their hearing; but contacts with service workers in these settings, unlike the nursing home, are brief and have relatively little impact on clients' lives.) At Crescent, there were times when conversations during patients' meals distracted aides and reduced the support offered. It was especially dehumanizing when aides talked unkindly about patients in front of them, as if they were not there, something that often happened in the dayroom as well as in casual meetings on the floor.

Jokes told at residents' expense, a regular feature of floor life, can be harmful, too. Admittedly, such shared humor is adaptive for aides. "We must laugh, we have to work here," Ms. Riley commented, after joking at lunch with her friends about patients who hit and scratched. In much the same way, Rebecka Lundgren and Carole Browner (1990) emphasize how shared humor about residents, built out of understandings of residents' limitations and idiosyncrasies, offered paid caregivers to the institutionalized mentally retarded a means to cope with demands of the job and provided needed emotional release.[1] In so doing, they argue, joking gave workers the reinforcement to offer empathetic care. Maybe so. But some of the shared humor I observed, occurring as it did in front of patients, often the ones who were the butt of the jokes, was cruel. Pressures operate to squelch criticism of such jokes. Because aides fear being chastised or isolated by co-workers, those who do not approve keep their feelings to themselves. Typically, they look the other way or simply smile weakly.

Fortunately, most of the aides' socializing occurs off the floor, away from the residents they care for. Meal breaks—on the day shift, a one-hour lunch and a fifteen-minute morning coffee break—are the highlight of the day. Usually, workers on a floor rotate first and second lunch. Some manage to always have their preferred lunch hour, and thus there is a small group of first-lunch and second-lunch regulars. Except for occasional trips to the nearby post office and bank, aides stay in the nursing home during lunch, no matter how nice the weather. A free meal is a perquisite of the job, and aides eat in the staff dining room, their turf, with a few venturing into the larger and brighter main patient dining room.

Ethnic clustering is a fact of life at lunch, although not a hard and fast rule. Because of lack of space but also sometimes by choice, workers from different ethnic groups often eat and talk together. As I mentioned previously, family as well as work concerns draw workers together and make for animated conversations. So do the soap operas broadcast during lunch, which a number avidly watched. A television set occupies a prominent place in the staff dining room, and there is an even larger one in the main patient dining room. Virtually all workers know the plots and characters in the favorite program, "All My Children," and there were cheers, claps, and hisses at especially dramatic moments.

Meals and breaks are a time for what Westwood (1985) calls "informal economics." A few workers have a lively trade selling cosmetics for Avon Products and other companies. Aides spend a lot of time looking at catalogs, discussing the merits of various products, and making purchasing decisions. The same workers who travel miles for bargains bought what I thought were overpriced jewelry and cosmetics from catalogs. They insisted that the products were superior, but I suspect other factors were at work. Buying products from co-workers cements social relationships, as I found out when I bought some items for my daughter. To continually say no to a co-worker who peddles a cosmetic line is to risk alienating her. There is, too, the convenience factor. And reciprocity is involved as well, since workers might, in the future, be hawking their own wares, including raffle tickets for churches or other organizations.

In fact, a number of workers used mealtime to sell candy and cookies for their children's schools. Many New York City public schools organize selling contests to raise money, with prizes going to the children who sell the most candy and cookies. One woman, eager to help her six-year-old son, made 110 sales in the nursing home, including sales to administrators and white-collar staff. Aides of all ethnic backgrounds spend the money, from $2 to $10, for the expensive cookies and candies. It is difficult to refuse a co-worker asking for help for her son or daughter; all workers highly value education for their children and want them to do well. I went out of my way to buy candy from mothers, which turned out to be important in developing and solidifying relationships with several aides.

There are also collections for sick workers. When an aide is away from work for more than a few weeks, invariably a friend or co-worker on the floor organizes a collection; most feel constrained to participate no matter what their relationship with the ill worker.

SUSUS AND BIRTHDAY CLUBS

Aides have also formed rotating credit associations on their own. These are groups with a core of participants who make regular contributions to a fund that is given to each contributor in rotation. Their presence at the Crescent Nursing Home reflects the heavily West Indian composition of the work force, since rotating credit associations flourish among West Indian immigrants (Bonnett 1980). Indeed, at Crescent, they are called "susus," a term used throughout the New York West Indian community.

On the day shift alone, there were four active susus and two birthday clubs during my stay. At any one time, more than half of the nursing aides belonged to a susu. Every Wednesday, on payday, workers sought out the organizer of their susu to pay their share, anywhere from $50 to $100 depending on the particular group. Each susu lasted from ten to twenty weeks; the pot was $500 to $1,500 depending on the number of participants and the amount given weekly.

Ms. Darius, a Haitian aide, formed her susu soon after moving from the evening shift to the day shift. She recruited fourteen nursing aides to give $100 a week for fifteen weeks. With her own share included, she collected $1,500 a week. Each participant picked a number, by lots, that determined the order of drawing the pot. The woman who drew number 1, for example, took out the entire $1,500 the first week of the susu; number 15 had to wait for the last week. The susu run by Denise Randall, an aide from Bermuda, was the longest-running in the nursing home, going strong for over twenty years. As constituted in spring 1989, it had fifteen participants and involved $50 a week, with a pot of $750.

These two susus were run by and made up almost entirely of nursing aides, with one or two West Indian clerical workers sometimes joining. They drew on black workers from different ethnic groups, each with a mix of Jamaicans, black Americans, and Haitians. The other two susus active during my research were run by Dominican men on the housekeeping staff. The members were virtually all Hispanic, including nursing aides as well as men in the housekeeping and dietary departments.

As soon as one susu was complete and all had, in nursing home parlance, "gotten their susu," another cycle began, usually with a few different participants, sometimes with a different amount per week as well. Denise's previous susu, which ended when I was beginning my research, involved twenty people, and the draw was $1,000.

The two birthday clubs on the day shift operated on the principle of shares: each birthday that a worker wanted to draw for was a share. Some had only one share, for their own birthday; others, who put in for their children, could have as many as four or five shares. Altogether, the birthday club run by Ms. Baker, a black American aide, had fifty-three shares; Denise's had forty-three. For each share, a worker owed $10 in any week there was a birthday. An aide with three shares in a birthday club owed $30 in a week when one member of the club had a birthday; in a "two-birthday week," she owed $60. In Denise's club, the amount taken out on each birthday was $430; in Ms. Baker's, $530.

Susus and birthday clubs offer the means and motivation to save money. They are particularly valuable to low-income workers who, given their limited economic resources, might easily spend all their earnings on daily household needs and consumption items. Many nursing aides planned to use their susu money for specific purposes; for example, one woman wanted to buy a washing machine, and another wanted to use it to pay for her daughter's tonsilectomy, which she chose to have done at a private hospital.

In the immigration literature, rotating credit associations are typically treated as "traditional" cultural institutions, brought over from the sending society and drawing co-ethnics together in their new home. Their role in facilitating capital accumulation for immigrant businesses is frequently emphasized and cited as an important reason that certain ethnic groups, from Koreans to West Indians, are successful in ethnic enterprises (e.g., Light 1972; Portes and Bach 1985).

Looking at rotating credit associations in the work place setting, rather than in the immigrant community, casts these groups in a somewhat different light. As far as I could tell, at the Crescent Nursing Home, rotating credit associations do not have anything to do with savings for business efforts. Far from being a "traditional," ethnically exclusive form, susus and birthday clubs have become part of the work culture of all low-skilled employees in the nursing home, bringing together workers from different ethnic groups. Indeed, the very term used at Crescent for rotating credit associations, "susu," has been adopted by workers of all ethnic origins, even though it is a West Indian (African-derived) phrase. Admittedly, Hispanic workers belong to Hispanic-run susus that have, with only a few exceptions, other Hispanic members. However, among the black work force, black Americans, Haitians, and English-speaking West Indians participate in the same susus and birthday clubs.

Whichever group aides join, participation in them gives workers a common bond. All the susus and birthday clubs operate according to the same basic principles. Perhaps most important, susus and birthday clubs are the workers' institutions, run by them and with no interference from higher-level administrative staff. Talk of susus and birthday clubs livens up the workday. A normal part of payday routine is giving one's payment to the organizer, and there are frequent discussions about where to locate her (or him). Birthday club participants always want to know how many birthdays are coming up, since this determines the amount they will have to put in. One afternoon in the staff dining room, when Ms. James eagerly told aides that there were five birthdays in the coming month, many began to calculate how much they would owe. Sometimes, more sensational news is part of the gossip stream, as when one aide's birthday money—the entire $430—was stolen in the nursing home.

Being informally selected as organizer or, as in Ms. Darius's case, successfully putting together a susu indicates that the person is trusted and respected by other aides. She is responsible, after all, for a sizable amount of money and for the details of record keeping and money collecting. Denise Randall explained, with pride, "[More than twenty years ago] this Spanish girl who ran it leave and tell me to take over. I say no and everyone say Denise you do it, you do it." Her susu is so well established that she does not have to do any recruiting. As she said, "People come to me."

Workers often thank the organizer by giving her "$10 or so" when they get their susus, although this is not a formal requirement. More important, being in charge of a susu or birthday club adds to the individual's prestige and puts her at the center of a large network of workers who come to her regularly, with trust, with their money. Of course, conflicts sometimes arise. One aide bitterly told me, "No more susu for me," because the man in charge embarrassed her publicly when she neglected to come in one payday, her day off, with her money.

On the whole, those in charge of a susu have an added sense of importance. When I think of susus at Crescent, I have a picture of Denise, notebook in hand, sitting at lunch amid a group of nursing aides, as she chatted and crossed off the names of those who had already given her their money that week. While she emphasized the burden of the work involved, she clearly enjoyed and felt proud to be doing her "other" important job.

HELPING ON THE JOB

A main tenet of the nursing aides' work culture is that they should help each other in caring for patients. In fact, aides often do give each other a hand. As a result, they have an easier time doing their job. Patients benefit, too, in that helping patterns often lead to better care and can even be said, at times, to increase "productivity."

As Gubrium (1975: 127–128) observed in his study of a midwestern nursing home, the informal assistance rule at Crescent is mostly confined to heavy care and what he calls "unruly" patients—those, in other words, whom workers have trouble handling alone at a particular time. Otherwise, aides are expected to do their own work. Since most patients at Crescent are in the heavy care category, aides frequently turn to each other for help.

Occasionally, aides need an extra hand to calm and restrain a screaming resident, but by and large, assistance is requested for everyday bed and body work chores. "I might need help getting up a patient," Ms. Ross said, "or in turning and positioning. And putting a patient in a wheelchair with the Hoyer lift and making sure they are comfortable." Working with heavy, immobile residents who must be moved limb by limb is less strenuous and less frustrating when two aides are involved. It is often safer, for both aides and patients. "You can damage a patient and damage yourself," said Ms. Darius, explaining why it was better to have assistance lifting certain patients. When no one else was around, she washed, changed, and made the bed of an extremely contracted, bedridden resident by herself; it took much less time and was much easier when another aide was available to help.

Requesting assistance is perfectly acceptable, as long as aides make it clear that such help is necessary and that they cannot manage alone. (This is unlike what Lundgren and Browner [1990] report in their study of the work culture at a state hospital for the mentally retarded. There, the unwritten rule was that workers should offer help without being asked; they felt uncomfortable asking for help.) On every floor at Crescent, aides regularly yell out to one another for help, calling the name of the particular worker they want. "If you need help," said one woman, summing up the ethic among Crescent aides, "you ask for it. We try to help each other. Some of them [patients] are very difficult to care for. If you need help, I will help you; if I need help, I'll call you."

Who helps whom is largely a function of proximity: aides in nearby sections tend to be those who give each other the most help. Personal likes and dislikes as well as ethnicity also play a role. Workers who do not get along obviously are loath to ask each other for help even if they work in adjacent sections. By the same token, workers who are friends—usually in the same ethnic group—will go out of their way to help each other, even if this means walking to the other side of the floor. Florence Wright, a black American woman, tried to explain how much Ms. Hill, a Jamaican aide on the floor, helped her. "The other day, Hill come and say something smelling awful in the hall by the elevator. Fisher [Florence Wright's patient] had a BM and I went and it did smell! Hill say, 'I'll run the water in the whirlpool,' and she bring the lifter for me and she say, 'I'll help you get caught up on your work.' She helped me put Fisher in the whirlpool bath and help me get it done."

Learning the helping ethic is part of socialization to informal floor rules. When I asked workers how they initially got accepted by other aides on their floor, a number mentioned that it was by conforming to the helping rule. "When they call you for help, don't refuse." Or as another worker put it, "If someone come and call and ask for help, I help." By the same token, many said that "not pitching in and helping" got nursing aides in trouble with others.[2] To consistently ask others for help but refuse to provide it in exchange is to violate the norms of reciprocity: generally other workers will feel no obligation to respond to their call. As Ms. Etienne told me, "If I call you, and you don't help, then when you call me, I won't help." To make sure I understood that she was not such an offender, she quickly added, "I'm just guessing; it never happen to me."

Other sanctions enforce the helping patterns: workers who refuse to help are sometimes criticized to their faces or behind their backs (cf. Lundgren and Browner 1990). As Gubrium (1975: 127) notes, eventually, an uncooperative aide is neither sought for nor given help and gains a reputation for being "hard to work with." By and large, the fear of these negative sanctions is effective.

Opposition and Resistance

The nursing aides' work culture does more than help them get along on the job. It also expresses their oppositional outlook and values (Benson 1986) as well as what some call "strategies of resistance" (e.g., Lamphere 1987; Shapiro-Perl 1984). Some scholars would even see elements of resistance in practices I have already described. Lamphere's analysis, for example, would suggest that the creation of ties among workers across ethnic lines, through savings associations and helping patterns, provides a potential basis for collective solidarity and action. Workers' informal conversations on patient floors, in violation of official regulations, if one follows Westwood's (1985) account, are a form of resistance to management controls and work discipline.

Other aspects of aides' work culture express, more clearly and more directly, opposition to management's authority and the conditions in which they work. Indeed, there are ways aides try to redefine and take some control over the work process.

On the face of it, this seems unequivocally positive for nursing aides. In line with the emphasis in the work culture literature, aides' resistance, we can say, shows that they are not passive players, resigned to difficult working conditions; rather, they are active agents who make choices, assert their interests, and try to determine their working conditions and challenge managerial authority.

But, in the nursing home, aides' opposition and resistance are more complex than in the factories that are typically described in work culture studies[3] or even in other service settings, like restaurants or stores, where care is not involved.[4] Like other service workers in "caring institutions," aides bear a special burden. For when aides "resist" or "oppose" management and assert their own interests, this is not always in the patients' best interests. Indeed, group pressure to assert informal control may pose problems for conscientious aides who want to offer good care.

RATE BUSTING

One of the most common resistance strategies mentioned in shop floor studies is the attempt by workers to determine how much they should do and to outwit employers' efforts to wring more production out of them (Montgomery 1979: 12). Frequently, workers establish output quotas among themselves or slow down their productivity as a way to resist the feverish pace and claim their own time. Also, there is the belief that if they turn in more work, employers' expectations and demands will go up or piece rates will be slashed (Burawoy 1979; Cooper 1987; Shapiro-Perl 1984; Roethlisberger and Dickson 1939).

Outside of the factory, in department stores in the early part of this century, Benson (1986) sees the enforcement of the stint as a way female clerks countered management's authority. As they approached the informal selling quota, clerks tapered off their selling efforts or retired to do stock work. "The worst sin the saleswoman could commit was to be a grabber: to ignore the stint and compete too energetically for customers" (Benson 1986: 248). Informal penalties awaited rate busters: ridicule and humiliation and, in extreme cases, social ostracism and exclusion from cliques. Physical reprisals also enforced the stint: messing up the offender's assigned section of stock or bumping into her (see Roethlisberger and Dickson 1939, on "binging," hitting a man hard on the upper arm).

At the Crescent Nursing Home, there are no unofficial quotas among workers and no deliberate slowdowns. Each aide has a set number of tasks to do for each assigned patient. Women who work during coffee or lunch breaks are not, as in the plant Westwood (1985) studied, stigmatized by co-workers. Usually, the only ones to forgo breaks (or part of the lunch hour) are slow workers who use this time to do required chores, like bed making, that they have not been able to finish earlier. "Rate busting" in the nursing home is mainly a matter of adding new tasks to the required list of assignments or responding to patient requests that are not viewed as part of the nursing aides' duties.

"A lot of people argue and say I'm not supposed to do this or that, and that's where there are difficulties," Ms. Roy told me. "When I started working here," she continued, "one of the patients asked me for some coffee. I went down to get it and one of the nursing aides said you better not do it because I'm not going to do it. And I said I'm gonna give her coffee; when she ask you, you just tell her no. And I still have this problem. I try to get candy for Martin and Rossini. Some people [aides] have this attitude; if you give, they say *they* will have to give."

Ana was accused of rate busting by a co-worker—"She say I do too much"—when she refused to use shortcuts devised by other aides to make certain tasks easier. "When you change a patient, you supposed to wash and grease them and she [the co-worker] don't do it. She say I take too long with mine." To avoid criticism and pressure to stint in ways she felt were unacceptable, Ana does not ask this other aide for help.

These examples highlight the special nature of rate busting in the nursing home. What in the factory is a resistance strategy against management, in the nursing home also has profound implications for patients. Doing what the work culture says is "extra" work to produce more bolts in a factory or to sell more dresses to affluent, transient department store customers is not the same as doing more for frail, dependent old people whom aides look after every day. To accede to group pressure in the nursing home, is, in these cases, to cut back on care. (That rate busting is so rare at Crescent suggests that the pressures are successful and, of course, that most aides do not want to make more work for themselves.) Rate busters are the very best aides; they are most concerned with patients' well-being and willing to violate group norms to help residents.

On the factory floor, workers fear that rate busters will lead management to increase its demands, and this is a concern for nursing aides, too. Service employees who do "people work" have an additional worry, that rate busters will "spoil" the clientele they serve, who will also increase *their* demands. This is a major concern in the nursing home, as the coffee incident with Ms. Roy indicates. If you get one resident coffee in the morning, then others will be asking, too. This is not an unrealistic worry for aides, who do not want to have to say no to yet another set of patient requests.

REPORTING

The informal rule against reporting co-workers to supervisors or administrators can be viewed as another form of worker resistance to management. At the Crescent Nursing Home, it has additional implications: it puts pressure on aides to tolerate mistreatment and abuses they observe.

In the classic study of the Hawthorne plant of Western Electric, researchers documented a "no squealing rule": operators should not tell a supervisor anything that would reflect adversely on an associate. Anyone who did was labeled a "squealer" (Roethlisberger and Dickson 1939: 522). Typically, squealers told supervisors that workers were wasting time, monkeying around, or not working fast enough. In the nursing home, where people, not machines, are involved, informing on co-workers usually means telling about the way they treat patients.

The no reporting rule operates primarily among workers on the same shift. I heard of quite a few cases in which aides reported problems to supervisors which they felt were caused by the earlier shift. (They did not name a particular worker, but the nurse could easily find out who on the earlier shift was responsible for that section of the floor or that patient.) Aides feel little loyalty to workers on other shifts, whom they rarely see and do not have to work with. Moreover, aides can be blamed for a problem, for example, a bruise or bad rash, that they notice and do not report when they first come to work.

On their own shift and on their own floor, reporting another worker is viewed as treachery. Adhering to the no reporting rule is seen as essential to getting along with aides whose help they need and whose friendship, or at least goodwill, is important. "Reporting, that's one thing I don't do," said Nina. "If I see something wrong, sometimes I might talk to the person, but I don't report them. That's not right."

The no reporting rule is especially hard on the most compassionate workers, like Ana, who truly have patients' interests at heart. She was upset that an aide on her floor did not, as she was supposed to, change her patients in the afternoon but left them wet all day. Nonetheless, she told me, "I don't talk; I don't get in trouble." On another occasion, I asked Ana what she would do if she saw an aide doing something wrong. "I don't tell nobody. If they ask, I say I wasn't in that section; I didn't see what happened."

A patient's sister once asked Ana about an incident she had heard about [from a patient] involving another aide mistreating her sister. "I just keep quiet. I say to her, 'Why don't you come and check it out yourself?'" Ana would not even mention names to me when she talked about cases of mistreatment. "Some people are cruel, but I keep my mouth shut."

TERRITORIALITY

As an astute patient-observer ironically put it, nursing aides follow the territorial imperative. Officially, they are responsible for their own section of the floor, with their own assigned patients. Aides will of course help co-workers who ask or who run into trouble; during meal breaks, when some workers are off the floor, they assume responsibility for the patients of aides who are away. It is another matter altogether when the patients of other workers ask for help. When this happens, aides are generally reluctant to offer assistance.

This is not what the administration had in mind when they formulated the rules. They expect aides to respond to the calls of any patient who clearly needs help. In obvious emergencies, aides will step in. But if they feel a patient can wait, for example, to be changed or to be taken to the bathroom, they will ignore the plea. In effect, they are drawing the line at how much work they will do by refusing to assume what they regard to be other workers' jobs. They feel justified, since, officially, they are not responsible for others' patients. Aides are attempting to control the work process; but patients can be the ones who suffer.

Mr. Stone, the patient-commentator on nursing home norms, half-jokingly told me, "You could be in your room calling out, 'I'm dying, I'm dying,' and they would pass by and say it is not their assignment." When Ms. Tate answered Mr. Wood's call and took him to the bathroom, she made it clear, as she sullenly went about her duties, that she was doing him an enormous favor, as he was not really her responsibility. Some nurses go along with aides' notions of territoriality as an efficient way to get things done: they want aides to complete tasks for their own patients, not to get distracted by other workers' patients' needs. Thus, when an on-call aide went to respond to a resident, who had spilled water all over herself and was sopping wet, the nurse told the aide, "Don't worry, she's not your patient."

The strong sense of territoriality can discourage aides who might want to intervene to help patients they feel are not getting adequate care. Unless two women are good friends and have a regular working partnership, in which they constantly help each other out, aides will be annoyed or openly angry if a co-worker, on her own initiative, takes an active role in their patient's care. Such intervention is deemed to be an unjustified infringement on their work territory and is often interpreted as criticism. One day, Ms. Roy helped a woman who was having trouble getting dressed even though the patient was not "hers." Ms. Roy explained, "I was told [by the woman's assigned aide] very firmly, 'Don't do that, that's not your patient.' I said to myself, when I'm old I hope there's a Ms. Roy around."

Although the noninterventionist ethic leaves patients with unsympathetic aides in the lurch, it is also true that it protects those with good aides—most patients in the facility. A worker who has cared for a patient for months, perhaps years, knows his or her likes and dislikes. Some are fiercely protective of their residents to the point of getting angry with and even speaking to workers who fill in when they are off and do not take good care of their patients.

WORKER CONSCIOUSNESS

Aides' opposition to management is not, of course, always a problem for residents. It is expressed in a number of ways that have little, or no, effect on residents and sometimes even positive implications.

Take aides' complaints about the administration. Aides are conscious of their shared interests as workers and that these interests pit them against the administrators and department heads who run the institution. Although the safety-valve analogy must not be overdrawn, the fact is that when aides complain about and vent their anger at management, they release at least some hostility that might otherwise be directed at patients.

Most feel that the administration overlooks their needs and does not give them the recognition they deserve. "We do all the work here, but they [management] don't recognize it," was a frequent complaint. An especially angry worker told me, "They treat the nurses' aides as the underdog. We, the underdogs, are the ones who take care of the place. Do you think they say thank you?"

As we saw in chapter 4, the administration is viewed, by and large, as the source of demands and directives that make life on the job difficult and that can impede aides' ability to offer decent care. Aides, feel, too, that management is more concerned with the well-being of patients than of the workers who keep the institution running.[5]

An offhand joke I heard at lunch one day highlights the widespread antiadministration feeling. Jocelyn Edwards, a Jamaican aide, complained that someone discarded the container of food she left in the floor refrigerator. Ms. Roberts immediately tossed off the line, "It was probably Stern [the administrator]," and all the aides at the table burst out laughing. Though the administrator obviously does not clean out the floor refrigerators, the joke reflects aides' belief that he shows little consideration for them—another example, in their view, of the way management mistreats and slights aides.

That the food thrown out was cooked in Jamaican style added to Jocelyn's bitterness. Ethnic and racial divisions heighten aides' antipathy to management. Like Mr. Stern, nearly all the top administrators and department heads are white Americans.[6]

Another bond uniting aides and other service workers against the administration is union membership. The Crescent Nursing Home is a union shop, and all aides are union members. Top administrators complain of the union's hold over aides and the complex disciplinary procedures that make it difficult for them to fire incompetent workers.[7] For their part, aides see the union as being too weak and having too little impact in improving their working conditions. When I came to the nursing home, aides had been working for nearly a year without a pay increase; when an agreement was reached to provide a retroactive lump sum payment, it was a while in coming. The wage increase aides did get, 4 percent, was lower than that won in the same period by another, more militant health care workers union in the city. No wonder aides were bitter that the union had not managed to do better. "I hardly notice it," is how one worker referred to the raise, a sentiment shared by her co-workers. To aides, the most important benefit of union membership is the union-administered health plan, a major reason that many stay on the job. Quite a few attended the free nursing aide classes at union headquarters, although hardly any had ever been to the monthly union meetings held there.

PARTIES: A WORLD APART

The opposition between aides and the administration stood out in parties and events designed, ironically, by the administration to foster commitment and identification with the nursing home, to boost work morale, and to reward workers for their service. During my research, there were three such events: a catered lunch for all employees after the facility passed the state survey inspection; the annual Christmas party; and a cabaret night for the entire nursing home staff.

In some New Mexican factories, Lamphere (1985; Lamphere, Zavella, and Gonzales 1993) argues that participation in company-sponsored picnics, clubs, and contests "co-opted" workers' organizational skills and helped to prevent the possibility of a strong women's work culture in resistance. This did not happen at the Crescent Nursing Home. There were few nonwork activities sponsored by management, and aides reluctantly participated, if they participated at all, in those that did occur. Indeed, these events and parties symbolized and reinforced the marked divisions—in occupation, authority, and race and ethnicity—between aides and administrators.

The survey party was a catered lunch, replete with Chinese food, pies, beer and soda, and music. Held to thank employees and to celebrate passing the state inspection, the lunch took place in the patient dining room, which was specially decorated for the occasion. The morning of the lunch, administrative staff excitedly prepared; aides, on the floors, were indifferent or mildly interested, and some even resented the intrusion on their lunch hour. Since the party overlapped with both the first and second lunches, aides on first lunch had to wait an extra half hour to eat. Those addicted to soap operas were upset by the interference with their television viewing. Most would have preferred to eat on their own turf, in their own dining room, in the routine manner.

Passing the state inspection was a source of jubilation to the administration but of much less concern to aides. To high-level staff, including supervisory nurses, it was important that their departments pass and not receive any negative citations. Their prestige and indeed their jobs were on the line. For aides, it did not much matter. Even if the nursing department was cited for several failures, individual aides were unlikely to be blamed, and their prestige did not hinge on the survey results. Aides viewed the survey as yet another intrusion in their working lives.

Having so little interest in the survey results, aides did not feel excited about celebrating. Nor did the party foster a sense of identification with the nursing home. Lower-level workers identify with each other, not with higher-level staff; they see their interests as opposed to those of the administration. Generally, they do not feel comfortable socializing with those above them in the occupational hierarchy who, outside the party context, give them orders and evaluations. This social distance is reinforced and intensified by the racial divide.[8] At the party, aides sat by themselves or in the case of Hispanic women, with Hispanic porters. When, by chance, aides found themselves seated at the same table as a white superior, they seemed ill at ease. In general, aides were not dominant at the party, and they were not as comfortable as when they set the tone and held sway, among themselves, in the staff dining room.

The "ritual of reversal," where department heads served food to employees, was a failure. Unlike rituals of rebellion in many non-Western societies, where subordinates are permitted to vent their hostility toward and assume the roles of superiors (e.g., Gluckman 1956), this role reversal offered no such outlet. It simply involved superiors taking on the menial role of servers, with subordinates required to graciously accept the "offerings." Far from being interpreted as a gesture of goodwill, many aides were suspicious of the administration's intentions. In fact, this "serving for a day" heightened the cleavage with the administration.

At the party, department heads, dressed in white aprons and chefs' hats, stood behind tables laden with food. They ladled out portions to employees, who passed from one dish to the next. The department heads were in good spirits, enjoying their role and the party. As they saw it, their serving role was an act of gratitude to the employees. Aides, however, did not think it an honor to be served by department heads. Indeed, the special arrangement emphasized that normally department heads did *not* serve. Because occupational roles at the party were so sharply delineated between servers and served, the aides' low position in the nursing home hierarchy was especially prominent. Some aides resented having to accept food from administrators they disliked and distrusted. "I'm not going to take food from her," one woman proclaimed, referring to the nursing administrator she detested. A few aides even interpreted the "serving role" as a ploy by the administration to prevent them from eating too much. Aware that the party was a dismal failure, the nursing home administrator decided, the following year, simply to give each worker $100 after the survey was passed.

Aides had to go to the survey party if they wanted to eat lunch. No such strings were attached to the Christmas party and cabaret affair. The Christmas party was scheduled during the evening shift, although it began early enough for day shift employees to attend at the close of their workday. The nursing home furnished drinks and music; employees brought food so that various ethnic specialties were represented. While a few aides cooked special dishes, like curried goat, most on the day shift only popped in for a few minutes and then went home. Evening shift aides stopped in briefly to have their dinner. As one nurse put it, the aides did not think of it as their party. Like the survey luncheon, aides were outnumbered by other workers, and the presence of so many white-collar staff, in particular, made them feel uncomfortable.

The cabaret, a semiformal affair held one weekday evening in the nursing home, provided entertainment and dinner for those who signed up. Invitations were put in every employees' paycheck envelope, but although the event was free, and there were many reminders, not one aide attended. Day shift aides did not want to wait around for several hours after work for the cabaret to begin; night shift workers did not want to come in early. Evening shift aides, on duty at the time, could not manage to put on the semiformal attire that was required. In any case, the cabaret was viewed as "their"—the administration's—party, not their own.

Ethnic Cleavages and Petty Squabbles

Strong as the bonds are that unite aides, at times, against the administration, there are also divisions among them. Ethnicity is the most important. Understandably, aides are drawn to workers who share their cultural understandings and customs, language, and identification with the same homeland. In some senses, one can speak of different ethnic cultures among aides—Haitian, Hispanic, black American, and, the most dominant numerically, Jamaican.

The small groups that socialize at meals and breaks are generally drawn along ethnic lines (cf. Bookman 1988; Lamphere 1987). In a typical lunch hour, most Jamaicans sit at a table in the staff dining room that they have informally appropriated (one aide even has her own unofficial seat); older Hispanic women, whose English is very limited, are across the room at "their" table; a few Haitians huddle together speaking Creole; and a couple of West Indians, one or two black Americans, and two younger Hispanic women who speak fluent English scatter, in ethnically mixed groups, among the remaining tables. Down the hall, in the patient dining room, most of the black American aides (and two female black American housekeeping workers) can be found, along with a few West Indian and Haitian regulars.

At meals, aides share food they have brought from home with women from their ethnic group. With their fellow Jamaicans or Haitians, they can lapse into patois or Creole, talk about visits to their home country, make jokes that hinge on common cultural understandings, and even, on occasion, speak disparagingly about other ethnic groups.

In general, aides' friends in the nursing home are from the same ethnic group. On the floor, women of similar ethnic background gravitate to each other and are most likely to be helping partners. Ethnicity determines patterns of association outside the nursing home, too. When aides told me which workers they visited, called, or met for parties or shopping jaunts, invariably it was those with the same ethnic background. Even the small groups of two or three who walk to the subway regularly after work each day are ethnically homogeneous.

In drawing some aides together, ethnicity, at the same time, distances others. Aides generally feel less comfortable with workers from different ethnic groups, and, in some cases, the language barrier makes communication difficult. Even when they work on the same floor, women with different backgrounds sometimes know little about each other's lives. I was astonished one afternoon when Ms. Marshall, a Jamaican aide, indicated she did not know where Maria Castillo, a Dominican woman, came from, although they had been working on the same floor for at least a year. (Maria's English, by the way, was excellent, and she was about the same age as Ms. Marshall.) The two happened to be sitting at the same table at lunch. Talk turned, as it usually does in such situations, to common bonds between them: children and children's schooling; the soap opera on television; and their shared immigrant background. Both commented that they did not like fish in New York, at which point Ms. Marshall asked, "Don't they make fish like this in Puerto Rico?"

Ethnic divisions, in themselves, do not cause interpersonal disputes among aides, but they make it more likely for tensions, rooted in other factors, to escalate. As in other communities with egalitarian norms, there is a strong sensitivity to insult—to real or imagined snubs or claims to superiority—among nursing aides (see Foner 1973; Jayawardena 1963). Petty jealousies and resentments and personality clashes also lead to hostilities. When women in the same ethnic group are involved, typically, they manage to work things out, or a mutual friend intervenes to settle the difficulty. When there is an ethnic divide between the disputants, this is less likely to occur. In fact, language and other cultural differences complicate and frequently heighten the tensions.

Tense relations with a co-worker can make life on the floor unpleasant for those involved and can add to the work burden. Ms. Price, a black American, and Ms. Braithwaite, a Jamaican, had barely been speaking to each other for months—"I say good morning to her and no more," said Ms. Price—even though they worked in adjacent sections. Neither asked the other for help, though this would have been most convenient. Nina, a young Dominican aide, described her relations with Ms. Roberts, a Jamaican, also in the next section. "We're like oil and water. We don't mix at all. She pick on me too much. Sometimes I say something and it bothers her. I don't know how she'll react. I stay away from her."

Hostilities as serious as these are rare. Because aides on the same floor have to work together day after day, there are pressures for rapprochement. There is a strong ethic of cooperation, of trying to get along despite underlying strains. Actual quarrels come and go. As one woman told me, "Sometimes they get on each other's back. But is like a family quarrel. One minute they fight, the next minute they friends. Sometimes they hate each other, but when they're together they talk."

Conclusion

The analysis of work culture in the nursing home shows that, on balance, co-workers are more help than hindrance. Without their companionship and physical assistance, many nursing aides would have trouble getting through the day. Despite grumblings about the difficulties of the job, for a great many aides, the Crescent Nursing Home has become, in some ways, a home away from home. Over the years, many have developed close relations with each other, ties that sometimes extend outside the bounds of the facility. Common understandings about work and about patients knit them together, as do various informal nonwork activities and involvements. There is also comradeship in adversity—shared complaints about management and residents that give them the sense that they are not alone in their frustrations. And although aides are cynical about the union, they know that unionization has brought wages and benefits that make them reluctant to leave the nursing home.

Less happily, aspects of the work culture that aides have forged pose problems for the most compassionate and most caring workers. Willing to go out of their way and beyond the requirements of the job to help patients, they can find themselves confronting group norms that discourage such efforts and pressure them to tolerate mistreatment. Moreover, quite apart from the work culture, the petty interpersonal conflicts that invariably arise among those who work closely together can, if they become serious, be another pressure point for aides.

In the end, as always, we return to the fortunes of patients, whose lives are so closely intertwined with those of their aides and who make the nursing home a special kind of work setting. For patients, too, as we have seen, the aides' work culture, coping strategies as well as resistance, has mixed effects. To the extent that the work culture sanctions neglect and cruel behavior, it does have a negative impact on patients. But this, of course, is only part of the picture. There is a brighter side, which must not be overlooked.

In the nursing home, informal practices that "manufacture consent" and enable aides to adapt to the job, from mutual assistance patterns to letting off steam at mealtimes, frequently benefit the "products" of aides' labor: patients. Indeed, it could well be argued that by helping aides keep up with their jobs, generally with good humor, the work culture, on balance, makes the nursing home a better place for residents.

8

Conclusion: Caregiving Dilemmas

Nursing home aides are overworked and underappreciated. Yet such characterizations are too simple to fully understand the difficulties they confront on the job and the many complexities, contradictions, and paradoxes in nursing home work.

Nursing aides face basic caregiving dilemmas. They are the ones who provide most of the direct patient care, and they are expected to do so with consideration and sympathy. The trouble is that structural features in the nursing home environment can militate against this kind of treatment. Nursing aides handle a complicated juggling act. As they try to do their job of looking after patients, they face pressures from numerous constituencies in the nursing home, each with its own needs and problems.

In analyzing these pressures, I have drawn on a number of theoretical perspectives and, in the process, have expanded them in light of the nursing home context. This includes elaborating theoretical approaches to contradictions in bureaucratic organizations, the links between the family and work place, the role of informal work cultures, and the place of gender among co-workers as well as in hierarchical relations on the job. In this final chapter, I touch again on a number of these issues as I summarize some of the central points about aides' caregiving dilemmas. I take a closer look, as well, at questions of race, ethnicity, and gender that have come up at different points in previous chapters. On a wider canvas, this study has implications for understanding the difficulties confronting other workers who provide services to people on the job. Ultimately, there is a question of whether the dilemmas nursing aides face are inevitable and whether changes are possible which could both lighten their burden and improve the lives of nursing home patients.

Understanding nursing aides' dilemmas is of more than academic interest. Nursing home aides are an expanding sector of the nation's work force. According to Department of Labor estimates, there will be an additional 350,000 aides in nursing and personal care facilities by the year 2005, bringing the total up to nearly a million.[1] And, of course, millions of Americans depend, in one way or another, on nursing home aides. Indeed, for better or worse, most of us will be closely involved with the nursing home world in our lifetimes, some of us as patients ourselves, others as relatives of those who live there.

Caregiving in the Nursing Home

PRESSURES AND CONTRADICTIONS

This in-depth study of one New York nursing home shows that aides are "women in the middle," subject to a barrage of contradictory pressures. Debilitated, ailing, and confused patients make ceaseless demands on aides. Patients' spouses and children, trying to look after and protect their relatives, often create additional pressures. So do nursing supervisors, themselves eager to get their work done and establish authority over their staffs. Administrators plague aides with rules and regulations designed to ensure decent care and the very survival of the nursing home. Co-workers, concerned to complete their own assignments, protect their bailiwicks, and limit their work loads, can be another source of strain. In the face of these myriad pressures, aides are sometimes abusive to patients, but at the Crescent Nursing Home, this was rarely a consistent pattern. Most were neither saints nor monsters; generally, they gave decent, many times supportive and sympathetic, care.

One of the most startling contradictions in nursing home life emerges from the operation of bureaucratic regulations. These regulations are, in a sense, a necessary evil. They are essential for administrative efficiency, especially given the complex requirements of modern medical care and state regulations. Critically, bureaucratic procedures reduce the potential for neglect and abuse of powerless residents. Yet the emphasis on bureaucratic rules has its costs. It can discourage aides from taking the initiative in responding to patients' needs and result in giving higher priority to the performance of physical tasks than the less tangible, less easily measured emotional work of caring.

In the end, rules protecting patients and preventing abuse can, at the same time, act as a brake on the very kind of supportive care administrators wish to foster. No matter how insensitive or cold, aides on some floors at Crescent were rewarded for completing their work efficiently and quickly; slower, more compassionate workers who violated regulations in an effort to help patients could find themselves the butt of the nurses' anger.

Another important contradiction involves what I call the paradoxes of resistance. In the nursing home, aides' work culture takes on special dimensions, adding new complexities to studies of resistance to management on the work floor. Informal strategies that Crescent aides developed among themselves to assert their interests and control over the work process—informal rules against rate busting, reporting, and interfering with other aides' patients—invariably affected patients, sometimes for the worse. There were cases in which devoted workers felt pressured to keep criticisms of co-workers' abuse to themselves, or in which they were under attack from other aides for going out of their way for patients.

PLEASURES AND STRATEGIES

The theme of this book is the dilemmas nursing aides face, but, we have also seen, their work brings pleasures, too. Aides at the Crescent Nursing Home carved out a bearable, often fairly satisfying work life, developing close relations with each other and sometimes patients as well. Although some workers are, as one aide put it, "just in it for the salary, just come and go," others deeply care. "If you're into it," the same worker told me, "you can really become part of the job and care for the people." Indeed, many aides received enormous satisfaction from looking after the helpless and needy elderly.

Work in the nursing home involves coping strategies to get through every day. The aides I knew improvised techniques to deal with and "get around" particular patients: learning their likes and dislikes; figuring out how to feed, bathe, and dress each resident efficiently and painlessly; and devising ways to cope with disruptive or abusive behavior. On the whole, aides worked out a modus vivendi with their nursing supervisors. The same was true for relations with patients' family members. And though they did not like the many regulations that constrained them, or many administrators in charge, mostly they gritted their teeth and toed the line because they did not want to risk losing their jobs and their benefits.

Then, too, despite the steady stream of rules, aides were able to establish a certain amount of autonomy on the floor. Although constrained by institutional rules and pressures, they were not, as one writer puts it in the context of psychiatric units, "swallowed up by the disciplinary agenda of the institution" (Rhodes 1991: 10). The nursing home sets limits on what aides can or cannot do, but there are "chinks and crannies" in disciplinary space in which they can recover the possibility of agency (ibid.). At the Crescent Nursing Home, aides were rarely under scrutiny as they went about the daily tasks of patient care. Within limits, they could control the pacing of the job, for example, which patients they chose to get ready first or how long they spent with each one. Although there were set procedures for each task, aides had some leeway as they tailored their techniques for individual patients. Moreover, if they were castigated by supervisors from above, the union offered strategies for job protection: disciplinary and grievance procedures spelled out in the union contract made firing workers extremely difficult.

The informal work culture Crescent aides shaped, outside the formal structure and rules of the institution, provided physical as well as emotional relief. Co-workers devised a system of mutual help that reduced the physical burden of patient care. And such practices as socializing at meals and the web of savings associations added an important dimension of sociability to the daily round of assignments and made work livelier and more interesting. Much as many aides would deny it, the fact is that Crescent had become, for a significant number, a kind of second home. Having worked together year after year, many aides formed close relations that often extended outside the bounds of the facility and even continued when they left the nursing home. Ms. Riley, one of the most disaffected aides I met, had nothing but negative things to say about the job when I knew her. Yet after she left to move to another state, one of the things she did on a trip back to New York was to visit the Crescent Nursing Home to see her old friends.

What is clear from this account is that aides' relations in the nursing home—with patients, supervisors, and patients' relatives—cannot be viewed in black-and-white terms. At times, patients were demanding and abusive; they could also become the objects of sincere affection and concern. Aides resented family members' interference, but a few workers became genuinely fond of certain patients' spouses and children. Some nurses were heartily disliked; others were admired and popular. A few aides often sincerely missed their former nursing supervisor when they moved to another shift. When Jocelyn Edwards first saw her former charge nurse (an LPN) after changing from evenings to days, she affectionately hugged her as the two sat down for a long chat. "This is my nurse," Jocelyn proudly told her friends. And while administrators generally were thought of in negative terms, there were a few of these, as well, whom aides respected and liked.

The Dynamics of Race, Ethnicity, and Gender

The nature and structure of nursing aide work and aides' responses play themselves out against the background of the social characteristics of the nursing home work force. As the nursing home industry grows, Diamond (1992: 186) observes, it builds off labor that has a distinct gender, class, and racial foundation. Aides in American nursing homes are overwhelmingly women and working class, and there is a steadily increasing number of minorities, especially in major urban areas like New York.

This composition of the work force has enormous implications for what goes on within nursing homes. From the aides' perspective, race and gender, as well as ethnicity, affect relations with those they care for, work with, and take orders from, sometimes providing a source of solidarity and sometimes accentuating divisions and dilemmas. Class comes into play mainly as it overlaps with occupational inequalities among staff. At Crescent, it had little bearing on relations with patients. Frail and dependent patients, often confused and sometimes comatose, were nearly always in reduced financial straits and had hardly any possessions with them. Their former class or occupational status was largely irrelevant to and very often unknown by the aides who cared for them. Ms. James's vicious comment about a high-level administrator captures this kind of leveling. "Soon he's going to be here and we will wash his behind and rub Vaseline on it and strap him into a chair." His administrative status, in other words, now a source of hostility, would no longer matter if he became a patient.

What does still matter, however, is race, something that remains visible, for all to see. Where aides are overwhelmingly people of color and patients and top administrators overwhelmingly white, race aggravates already existing divisions. As a *New York Times* story puts it, the dramas of a city stratified by color play out every day in the nursing home (Fisher 1993). Racial differences feed into and intensify, rather than create, divisions between groups in the nursing home. At Crescent, they added to the aides' sense that patients, as a group, were in an opposite camp and increased antagonism to management as well as social distance from patients' relatives.

The impact of race on patient care clearly calls for further study. My impression, at Crescent, is that aides did not treat minority patients any better than those who were white. Even aides with minority patients usually had white patients as their special favorites. Racial epithets were deeply stinging, but they were hardly the only form of abuse workers had to endure from residents, and despite the small number of minority residents, a couple were truly disliked by their aides. What we obviously need are systematic studies comparing aides who tend to patients of the same race with aides whose patients are of a different racial background.[2]

Ethnicity must figure in these comparisons, too, for, within racial categories, ethnic differences can be an important basis of separation. And not just from patients. Much as ethnicity brings some aides together, it divides others. I would not go so far as to characterize the Crescent work place as made up of "existential worlds of ethnic isolation," a phrase Guillermo Grenier and Alex Stepick (1992) apply to the Miami construction site and apparel plant they studied. Yet Crescent aides mainly socialized with and preferred to lend a helping hand to co-workers in the same ethnic group, and it was easier to patch up differences with them as well.

A further complicating factor is gender. Like race, it is a tie that, among aides, can help bridge ethnic divisions. As women and mothers, aides at Crescent shared interests, concerns, and worries that gave them a sense of common cause and helped underpin and give a distinct tone to their work culture. Motherly concerns, as well as troubles with men, occasionally strengthened links between aides and some of the more alert female residents. In much the same way that popular nurses drew on racial and ethnic identities they shared with aides, they could also build on common womanly interests, symbols, and styles to nurture good relations with aides.

Yet shared gender roles and identities, in themselves, did not ensure cooperation or overcome wide inequalities of status and power among female staff in the nursing home. What stood out at Crescent was how keenly aides felt—and so often resented—the authority of coordinating and administrative nurses. High-level female staff issued orders and were in charge and in a number of subtle and not so subtle ways emphasized their superior status to aides. Not surprisingly, in the nursing home work place, occupation was of overwhelming importance in shaping relations among staff. Among "occupational equals" like nursing aides, common gender and racial identities and, in some cases, common ethnicity served to reinforce bonds that had already developed on the basis of shared interests and problems on the job.

Are Nursing Home Aides' Dilemmas Unique?

As a study of nursing home aides, this book, understandably, has documented the special nature of nursing home work, its rewards, problems, and idiosyncrasies. But if the burden of caring for weak, ill, and often demented elderly nursing home patients is in some ways unique, in others it is not. Nursing home aides share dilemmas with other low-skilled workers, especially those, like themselves, employed in caregiving institutions. Looking at nursing aides' dilemmas in a larger, comparative context not only highlights some of the special aspects of their jobs but also helps to better appreciate the constraints and difficulties of other Americans who do "people work." Given the enormous growth of service sector jobs in the American economy, this analysis is especially relevant. Theories of work in Western societies have largely been shaped by studies of industrial labor, and it is time to revise and expand these views in light of the increasingly important service occupations.

HUMAN SERVICE WORK

People work inevitably brings stresses and strains that those who work on products and objects do not experience. Goffman (1961: 74–80) noted many of these difficulties in his classic study of total institutions. Because "human materials" can become objects of fellow feeling and even affection, sympathetic staff will suffer if they have to inflict hardships. People, unlike inanimate objects, can purposely and intelligently thwart staff plans. And staff must often take into account the statuses and relationships that the people they "work on" have outside the work setting.

The difficulties Goffman mentions are especially acute for workers, like nursing home aides, whose contact with "inmates," "clients," or "patients" is continuous and long-lasting. Even service workers, like sales clerks, waitresses, and flight attendants, who deal with the public and whose jobs involve what Hochschild (1983) calls emotional labor, have transitory interactions with those they serve. Whereas a waitress or store clerk has to cope with rude or rowdy customers, they soon go away. Disruptive patients remain day after day—in nursing homes, sometimes months and years. Unlike people work in offices, stores, or restaurants, the family enters nursing homes and hospitals in the form of relatives of patients who, we saw, bring with them their own set of demands and pressures—kin as critics, in Goffman's (1961) phrase.

As these comments suggest, nursing home aides have most in common with nonprofessional "people workers" in institutions designed to offer care, that is, human service organizations like hospitals, social service agencies, and health clinics.[3] Industrial laborers, standing by their machines, and clerical workers, sitting at their computers, are not expected to offer care as part of their jobs. Paid caregiving often involves the expression of genuine feelings, not, as in many other kinds of service work, like the flight attendants Hochschild (1983) describes, simply the marketing of affect.

Because people workers in human service organizations often sincerely want to help those they care for, the work cultures that develop among them pose a dilemma that "object workers" do not face. Workers may find themselves caught between the demands of co-workers, on the one hand, and the demands of clients or patients, on the other. As we saw at the Crescent Nursing Home, informal customs and practices that allow human service workers to assert control and resist management can, at the same time, hinder the efforts of conscientious employees to provide the kind of care they would like. The pressures from co-workers to refrain from reporting negligence or doing extra work were relatively mild at Crescent. They may be more severe in settings in which workers are subject to fewer regulations and less supervision (see, e.g., Scheff 1961, on a state mental hospital in the 1950s).

In human service jobs, statuses that workers and clients occupy outside the organization also shape the dynamics and difficulties of work. Emily Abel and Margaret Nelson (1990: 15–16) argue that when higher-status workers provide care to working-class and minority clients, caregiving shades easily into social control. When minority workers from working-class backgrounds, as in many nursing homes, deliver care to mainly white, middle-class clients, caregiving tends to embody significant elements of personal service. In such cases, workers run the risk of racial abuse or slurs from patients and condescension from patients' relatives. In the nursing home, where patients' former occupational or class status no longer means much in their present dependent condition, aides also exercise some degree of control. At the same time, workers' relations with administrators and high-level managers tend to reproduce class and racial inequalities in the wider society. As at the Crescent Nursing Home, those in top roles in the institution are often white and higher in the class hierarchy than those doing the actual caregiving.

Although gender inequalities may also be reproduced on the job and exacerbate workers' difficulties with clients and supervisors, this was not much of a problem at the Crescent Nursing Home, or, I suspect, at many other nursing homes. More so than most other human service organizations, nursing homes are predominantly female worlds. In all occupational fields, most paid caregivers are women, a reflection of the widespread cultural belief that caring is a "natural" activity for women. But in nursing homes, most patients are also women, and so are the aides' immediate supervisors on the nursing staff. At Crescent, even some of the high-level administrators were women. Typically, in nursing homes, top administrators and physicians are male, yet they are usually distant figures for aides and of little significance in their daily working lives.

The strains arising from the contradictions in bureaucratic organization create a critical dilemma for employees in human service institutions. In all bureaucracies, workers are likely to resent regulations that restrict their autonomy and supervisors who enforce the rules. In human service organizations, there is an added complication: a tension between regulations and standardized techniques, on the one hand, and the need for flexibility in attending to the needs of individuals, on the other. This tension stands out in people-sustaining organizations, such as nursing homes, where there is a pressing need for set procedures and universal criteria to minimize the potential for neglect and abuse of disabled, dependent, and debilitated clients (Hasenfeld 1983: 139).

As Abel and Nelson (1990: 12) aptly put it, caregiving fits uneasily into bureaucracies. Bureaucratic institutions operate on the basis of a set of general rules, but the essence of caregiving is attentiveness to the individual. The problems stemming from the rationalization of affective care may be especially acute for workers in health care settings like nursing homes, where dealing with patients' physical needs and meeting state regulations are given priority over the emotional components of care.[4]

CHRONIC CARE WORK: NURSING HOMES AND PRIVATE HOMES

A look at workers who perform the same tasks as nursing aides do but in private homes makes a fascinating comparison. For if nursing home aides suffer, in their eyes, from problems of overregulation, home care workers who see to the needs of the frail elderly can have difficulties precisely because the rules are not clear-cut.

By now, there are perhaps as many as half a million home care workers. Their numbers have expanded at a rapid rate with the growing number of chronically ill and disabled elderly and the search by state governments for ways to cut expenditures on long-term care (Feldman 1993; Feldman, Sapienza, and Kane 1990).

Like nursing home aides, home care workers must deal with physically demanding clients, who may be angry or abusive, as well as with interference from family members. Yet the dilemmas facing health care workers in private homes are very different from those in institutions. In New York City and throughout the United States, home care workers' hourly wages are lower, their benefits much less generous, and their jobs less stable than those of nursing home aides (see Burbridge 1993; Feldman, Sapienza, and Kane 1990; Cantor and Chichin 1990; MacAdam 1993). On their own, often with only a client for company, they receive none of the support or companionship from co-workers that makes work in a nursing home more bearable.

Nor do they experience the kind of bureaucratic constraints that plague aides at the Crescent Nursing Home, where nearly every aspect of their job is subject to some rule or order. For home care workers, the problem is that their duties are often ambiguously defined: it is unclear exactly what they are supposed to do. Conflicts can arise when a client or relative expects the worker to do things, such as the family laundry, that the worker feels are not part of the job. Another example: the care plan may call for a worker to prepare the client's lunch but not indicate whether the spouse's meal should also be provided (Eustis, Fischer, and Kane 1991; Cantor and Chichin 1990). When tasks are described generally, it may be hard for a worker to refuse.

Home care workers also have problems with unclear accountability, exactly the reverse for their counterparts in nursing homes. At the Crescent Nursing Home, the chain of command was all too clear to aides. The coordinating nurse is the pivotal figure through whom most problems, requests, and suggestions have to be cleared. A home care worker may have four or five parties—a nurse supervisor, an agency staff person, a case manager, a client, a member of the client's family—to whom she feels accountable and who may have different expectations for her (Eustis, Fischer, and Kane 1991).

As we have seen, in the nursing home, aides were frustrated by their inability to take the initiative and make independent decisions about patient care. The best aides felt their patients suffered as a result. In private homes, workers have much more autonomy in meeting the client's needs, but this can create dilemmas for workers when they do not have enough information on which to base their work. Home care workers have only limited contact with their agency supervisors; over half in a New York City study saw their supervisor less than once a month (Cantor and Chichin 1990). Conscientious home care workers often look for more, not less, supervision and guidance so they can do what is right for their clients. As an example, Nancy Eustis and her colleagues (1991) recount the frustrations of a worker who was not told exactly how to care for her client, who had radiation sores from treatment for breast cancer.

The informality that is a hallmark of home care is also problematic. Working one-on-one with clients, they can give more time to them and be more attentive to their needs than nursing home aides, who feel rushed as they move from one patient to another. Yet the intensity and informality of the personal relationship with clients create dilemmas. If a worker cannot be firm with her client and place boundaries on the relationship, there is a risk of exploitation—something that is more likely if there is any ambiguity about the tasks she is supposed to do (Eustis and Fischer 1991). Home care workers often work extra hours for which they are not paid, sometimes because they feel sorry for clients who need help or because they are reluctant to leave work unfinished (Cantor and Chichin 1990). As we saw, this almost never happened at the Crescent Nursing Home, where aides stopped work when their shift was over and rarely put in extra time without pay.

For home care workers, then, the dilemmas of ambiguous authority, unclear rules, and informality stand in stark contrast to the problems of rigid regulations facing aides in nursing home bureaucracies. It should be noted that whichever job is more difficult, the fact is that most, at least in New York City, would take the nursing home position if given the choice. Indeed, many aides at Crescent had, earlier in their careers, cared for the elderly in private homes; they viewed their present jobs as a definite improvement. For women struggling to support their families, the better wages and benefits in nursing homes ultimately take higher priority than the problems involved in caregiving on the job.

Are Caregiving Dilemmas Inevitable?

What this account makes clear is that the dilemmas nursing aides experience are not random or haphazard. They stem from the structure of the institution in which they work and the system of relations generated within it. The analysis in this book raises a vital and disturbing question: are the pressures discouraging compassionate care an inevitable product of forces in the nursing home environment, or are they amenable to change?

Each nursing home is, of course, unique, with a peculiar blend of policies, practices, and personnel. One can say, with Joel Savishinsky (1991: 257), that every nursing home has its own way of life or culture, shaped by, among other things, its size and financial base, location and architecture, background and health status of patients, and goals, hierarchies, and support systems of the staff. Partly because the Crescent Nursing Home is such a good one, with administrators intent on improving the facility's quality and passing state inspections with flying colors, the burden of regulations on aides was particularly heavy. Aides in less well run and less humane institutions probably have more autonomy, though, at the same time, there is also likely to be more serious and more frequent patient neglect and abuse. Elsewhere, wage and work load issues are much more of a problem for aides. Where aides' wages are appallingly low, barely above the minimum wage in facilities in some states and cities, the problem of poor pay obviously stands out in a way it does not at Crescent. And heavier patient loads in many places make it more difficult for aides to offer decent care (see Diamond 1992). Yet despite each facility's distinctive traits, the caregiving dilemmas identified at the Crescent Nursing Home are, I suggest, present to a greater or lesser degree in most nursing homes in this country.

Unfortunately, many of the pressures or dilemmas aides face come with the job and will not go away. Nursing home patients everywhere are increasingly ill and, inevitably, demanding and sometimes abusive. Aides could be more responsive to patients' needs if they had fewer residents to look after, in the best of all worlds, one or two apiece. However, much smaller patient loads are highly unlikely given the financial constraints that even nonprofit institutions confront. Patient-aide ratios like those at the Crescent Nursing Home, or even higher, are doubtless a given with which aides have to contend. On a case by case basis, social workers can work with especially troublesome family members to make them sensitive to the needs and problems of aides, yet relatives' frequent presence, in itself, is likely to lead to a certain amount of interference and escalation of care demands that aides, as they know, have to learn to live with.

Government-mandated regulations will not disappear. Nor, on the whole, would it be in the patients' interest if bureaucratic rules developed to regulate the way aides provide care were less strictly enforced. Most decisions related to caregiving procedures cannot be left to nursing aides because this opens the door to potential mistreatment and abuse. Nor will the nursing hierarchy go away either. Professional qualifications and pay inequities, to say nothing of the need for supervision on patient floors, invariably lead to inequalities among nursing staff. There are inherent structural conflicts when nurses have the authority to supervise aides and enforce management rules. As in most work environments, a co-worker culture is also bound to flourish among aides. Mostly, this is for the good; the work culture helps aides cope with their jobs and with patients. The negative consequences of the work culture are, I think, relatively minor compared to the benefits. In any case, management cannot force aides to report each other, and attempts to do so would seriously hurt worker morale.

If many of the pressures aides experience are inevitable, there are some possibilities for intervention and change that could ease the aides' burden and, at the same time, encourage good care. Let me mention just a few. Compassion cannot be legislated or charted, but it can be rewarded. More emphasis on the emotional side of care, at every level of the nursing home, combined with a system of rewards for sympathetic aides who go out of their way for patients can help combat pressures from administrators, nurses, and co-workers that discourage the best aides.

Admittedly, bureaucratic regulations encourage supervisors to praise rule following that produces readily measurable results. But nursing homes, in particular, nursing departments, should make conscious efforts to stress the emotional, as well as the physical, aspects of caring. In terms used in the nursing home literature, this means more of a psychosocial model of organization, with attention to the social and psychological needs of patients and less emphasis on a medical model and its stress on health problems that need diagnosis and treatment (Kane and Kane 1978; Johnson and Grant 1985).

Although the Crescent Nursing Home has incorporated much of the psychosocial model of care into its organization, with, among other things, a case management approach that includes both health and social services, more is needed. On patient floors at Crescent, nursing supervisors in charge talked endlessly to aides about the mechanical aspects of the job, but they almost never mentioned the psychological side. Nurses did not advise aides of ways to be kinder or more humane, nor did they criticize blatant cases of psychological mistreatment that occurred right before them. Nurses, who set standards for their floors, were themselves sometimes abusive to patients.

To ameliorate some of these problems, senior nursing staff, for one thing, need to be good role models for the aides they supervise. It is counterproductive if nurses ignore residents, spend little time with them, ridicule them, and fail to attend to their needs (Aroskar, Urv-Wong, and Kane 1990: 284). Administrators have to make clear that psychologically abusive behavior from nurses, which at the Crescent Nursing Home was open for all to see, is unacceptable. In-service training, for all nursing staff, that stresses sensitivity and emotional aspects of caring can also help. The Crescent administrator spoke to me of the need for such a course, best taught, he felt, by someone from outside the nursing home, about whom staff had no preconceived notions and with whom they had no earlier antagonisms. Because aides are concerned that in-services disrupt their routine and the work they could instead be doing, he thought that this course should, ideally, be offered after work and that aides should be paid overtime for attending. Even if financial constraints rule out outside instructors and overtime pay, innovative techniques would help capture the aides' attention; one example the administrator suggested was putting physical restraints on aides so they would experience how residents feel.

Also in order is training and encouraging nursing supervisors to praise compassionate care and to work with aides in devising ways to deal with difficult patients. Behavior like Ms. James's, described in chapter 4, cannot go without criticism. Certainly, she should not have gotten the highest ratings in her evaluations or special privileges as the nurse's pet.

By the same token, official rewards to sympathetic aides would send a clear message about what is important in care. Obviously, competence in the physical tasks is important, but the emotional work of caring—too long invisible and unnamed in nursing homes (Diamond 1990: 176)—must be given more consideration in the formal evaluation and reward structure. Perhaps, as a social worker at Crescent mentioned to me, it would even be well to give higher priority in these rewards to chatting, laughing, and developing good relationships with residents than to meeting every physical task to perfection. Better to have a patient a little messy but less depressed because aides have built up good relationships with them. An aide like Ana Rivera, conscientious, warm, and truly caring, should be praised and encouraged, not punished for the "sin" of going a bit slow.

Beyond praise and good evaluations, other signs of recognition can signal what is valued in care and, at the same time, perhaps make aides feel better about and take more pride in their jobs. In the good homes V. Tellis-Nayak (1988: 143) and his colleagues observed, aides were constantly written up in newsletters, their photos posted on bulletin boards, and awards routinely given to publicly toast the employee of the week, month, or year. What these awards were he does not say, but, more than honorary certificates, monetary prizes would be especially meaningful. Rewards to aides who are willing to help patients above and beyond the call of duty would also help counteract the pressures from co-workers to avoid performing "extra" work.

While the stresses and strains of the nursing aide job cannot be eliminated, coping mechanisms that are part of the official structure of the institution can help reduce their impact. One possibility, suggested in Savishinsky's (1991: 163–164) study, is a time-out room where aides can get away for a few minutes when the pressures are too much. Such a refuge would help aides calm down when residents hit, strike out, or curse them. As a nurse in the facility Savishinsky (ibid., 164) describes said, "When you can't strike back or run off, how do you keep your sanity, your self-respect?" Another formal coping mechanism, suggested in the same study, is a support group for staff where, at a set time, they could let off steam and discuss their anger at patients (ibid.).

Is More Autonomy for Aides Possible?

Bureaucratic demands may be an inevitable part of modern nursing homes, but must they constrain workers' autonomy and control to the extent that I found at the Crescent Nursing Home? Would it be possible to allow aides more autonomy without harming—indeed, perhaps helping—the patients?

The elaborate set of rules in place at the Crescent Nursing Home meant that aides had little ability to take initiatives in patient care. Not professionally trained and working with seriously ill patients, aides were not permitted to independently alter care plans or make decisions about medical treatments. Yet at the same time, they were the staff who spent the most time with patients and were most attuned to changes in their physical and emotional states.

This inability to exert control over the decision-making process was a source of frustration for some of the best workers at the Crescent Nursing Home and at times had negative consequences for patient care. Recall the case of Ana Rivera who, after making numerous requests to her coordinating nurse for a more comfortable hand protector for a patient, met with no response. When she finally ordered the glove on her own, she was severely castigated, and the glove was returned. In this case, the nurse's emphasis on bureaucratic procedures at the expense of patient welfare was extreme.

What this case highlights is the need for legitimate channels for aides who feel frustrated when they want to help residents and ways to involve aides in the care planning process. "Involvement" is the key word here. I am not arguing that aides should be allowed to act as independent agents. Even with the best intentions, this might cause patients real physical harm. I am not exempting Ana either. Although the glove she ordered would have helped the patient, similar kinds of independent action in other cases might be inadvisable from a medical or therapeutic perspective.

When nurses in charge ignore aides' suggestions or reports about problems with patient care—whether from intransigence, overwork, or heartlessness—aides should feel free, indeed, should be encouraged, to go above their immediate supervisor to the next level of authority. If such norms become established and the threat of "going above their heads" becomes real, nurses may well feel pressure to be more responsive to aides' concerns (Kjervik 1990: 207).

Although aides' input can be invaluable, too often in nursing homes everywhere, their opinions are ignored or never even solicited when designing resident care plans (Aroskar, Urv-Wong, and Kane 1990: 284). Informally, nurses and other professionals should be encouraged to ask aides what they think when problems arise with their patients (ibid., 286). A formal way to give aides a say in the decision-making process is to include them in treatment care conferences (something not done at Crescent) where they can hear the rationales for various professional decisions and make suggestions (Kjervik 1990: 203). Another possibility is to create what is known as primary assignments. In addition to their regular assignments, each day and evening shift aide would become the facility expert on one or more residents—medically, psychologically, and socially—and represent the resident's interests with other staff. In one nursing home where this practice was put into effect, morale among aides improved (Aroskar, Urv-Wong, and Kane 1990: 285).

Admittedly, these kinds of changes would not completely solve the problem of aides' lack of autonomy. And each suggestion has its own potential problems. Even if administrators make plain that aides can go above nurses' heads when their reports on patients are ignored, many will be reluctant to anger their immediate supervisors by taking such actions. Encouraging nurses to consult with aides about patient problems does not mean they will do so. Requiring aides to attend treatment care conferences or making additional primary care assignments, for many aides, will seem like simply another burden rather than a way to make their voices heard. Yet these suggestions make clear that more autonomy and control for aides are possible within the bureaucratic framework of the nursing home. Certainly, they are worth a try. Indeed, I think the changes will be most appreciated by the truly caring and supportive aides who want more say in patient care so they can improve the lives of the residents they look after.

Whether we like it or not, nursing homes are, for the foreseeable future, here to stay. Although alternative long-term care arrangements are bound to become more widespread, the medically unstable elderly or those in vegetative states, without relatives to oversee home care, are likely to spend some time in a nursing home. Clearly, our sympathies and concerns should be with the situation of the patients—frail, fragile, helpless, and all too often without advocates to speak for them. But we must not overlook the plight of nursing home workers, in many ways the unsung heroines of their institutions.

Through an in-depth analysis of workers in one New York facility, this study has portrayed the worlds of nursing aides and the dilemmas they grapple with in providing care. To those ready to blame aides for all the problems in nursing homes, I hope this account will, at the least, offer a sobering corrective. For most people reading this book, the possibility of becoming a nursing home patient or having a loved one admitted is a real and frightening prospect. The chances of working in a nursing home as an aide are remote. Yet in thinking about nursing home care we would do well to try to put ourselves in the workers', as well as the patients', place and ponder a question an aide I knew asked: "Now that you see our job, would you like to do this work?"

Notes

1: Introduction

1. Nursing aides and orderlies constituted over 40 percent of all full-time employees in nursing and related care homes in 1985 and 71 percent of all nursing staff (Strahan 1987).

2. The question of nursing aide turnover has come in for a lot of attention (Grau et al. 1991; Halbur 1982; Halbur and Fears 1986; Knapp and Harissis 1981; Schwartz 1974; Stryker 1981; Wallace and Brubaker 1982; Waxman, Carner, and Berkenstock 1984). Other topics that have been explored include mistreatment and encouragement of dependency among patients (Fontana 1977; Kayser-Jones 1990; Pillemer and Moore 1989; Sperbeck and Whitbourne 1981; Stannard 1973; Vesperi 1983); the nature of and attitudes toward work duties (Aroskar, Urv-Wong, and Kane 1990; Brannon, Streit, and Smyer 1992; Chappell and Novak 1992; Gubrium 1975; Henderson 1981); and attitudes to patients and the aged generally (Chandler, Rachal, and Kazelskis 1986; Gilliland and Brunton 1984; Kahana and Kiyak 1984; Lerea and LiMauro 1982; Penner, Ludenia, and Mead 1984; Sheridan, White, and Fairchild 1992; Wright 1988). An annotated bibliography of material on geriatric nursing assistants (Weber 1990) has a social work and practice-orientation slant; most of the 200 or so entries refer to training, organization development, evaluation, and advocacy.

The few qualitative studies that have nursing aides as their focus consider only some of aides' difficulties (Bowers and Becker 1992; Diamond 1988, 1990, 1992; Tellis-Nayak and Tellis-Nayak 1989).

3. These ethnographies are Diamond (1992), Gubrium (1975), Kayser-Jones (1990), Savishinsky (1991), and Shield (1988). Diamond's (1992) account does focus on nursing aides as well as patients. Based on his own experience as a nursing aide in three Chicago area nursing homes, he offers a

sympathetic portrayal of aides and a view of their daily work tasks, although he deals with only some of aides' dilemmas. It should be noted, too, that Gubrium (1975) devotes a chapter in his book on Murray Manor to the basic work routines of nurses and aides. Although Savishinsky's (1991) recent ethnography is subtitled *Life and Work in a Nursing Home*, his two chapters on staff focus on professional staff—a nurse, a social worker, a physical therapist, and an administrator.

4. The use of "Ms." was not a feminist strategy. Ms. was a neutral term that did not call attention to a woman's marital status, a status deemed unimportant among co-workers. Quite a number of aides lived with men without being married or were simply on their own with their children.

2: Setting the Context: The Nursing Home World

1. The figures are even higher—19,100 nursing homes with 1.6 million beds—if we add the nursing homes and board and care facilities not certified to accept Medicaid and Medicare payments (Strahan 1987).

2. The government directly pays about half of the total bill for nursing home care, mostly through Medicaid. Medicaid is financed jointly by federal and state governments and provides medical insurance for the indigent (of all ages), including unlimited nursing home benefits for those who qualify. Medicare provides national health insurance for the elderly through the Social Security program; during most of my research, in 1989, when the short-lived Medicare Catastrophic Coverage Act was in effect, Medicare paid for 150 days of nursing home care per year. With the repeal of the act, nursing home benefits paid by Medicare were again reduced, in 1990, to a maximum of 100 days of posthospital care if certain conditions were met. Given the way policies change, let me emphasize that when I use the present tense to describe government health funding programs, I refer to the time of the writing.

3. The national average age of nursing home residents in 1985 was 79, up from 78 in 1977. As for their physical state, the average number of ADL (activities of daily living) dependencies for residents increased from 3.5 in 1977 to 3.9 in 1985. (These dependencies include requiring assistance in bathing, dressing, using the toilet, transfer, eating, and difficulty in bowel and/or bladder control.) Mental disorders are also increasingly prevalent. In 1969, 11 percent of the nation's nursing home residents had a primary diagnosis involving mental disorders. By 1985, the figure was 22 percent. Sixty-six percent of the nation's nursing home residents were reported to have one or more mental disorders in 1985 (Hing 1989).

4. Prior to 1986, New York State paid facilities a set daily rate for each day of care given to Medicaid residents. This rate was derived from past costs with increases to allow for inflation. There were only two classes of rates: one for a skilled nursing facility (SNF), providing the highest level of nursing care, and one for a health-related facility (HRF), providing a lower level of care. Care

for all Medicaid residents at each SNF was reimbursed at the same rate; care for all Medicaid residents at each HRF was reimbursed at the same rate (Rudder 1988).

5. Personal communication, Robert E. Burke, project director, Multi-State Nursing Home Care Case-Mix and Quality Demonstration.

6. The 1987 Nursing Home Reform Act eliminated, as of 1990, the distinction under Medicaid between skilled nursing facilities and intermediate care facilities; all Medicaid-certified facilities are now required to have at least one registered nurse on duty eight hours a day, seven days a week and a licensed nurse (RN or LPN) on duty at all times. However, states may waive the nursing staff requirements if a facility can show "diligent but unsuccessful efforts to recruit the required personnel." For a useful summary of the 1987 Nursing Home Reform Act, see Coleman (1991).

7. Unless otherwise noted, all figures for the Crescent Nursing Home, including patients and staff, refer to the period during which I did my research.

8. Nationwide, 72 percent of nursing home residents are women, 92 percent are white, and 61 percent are widowed (with another 26 percent divorced, separated, or never married) (Hing 1989).

9. In 1989, when the Medicare Catastrophic Coverage Act was in effect, 81 percent of the patients at the Crescent Nursing Home were covered by Medicaid, 13 percent by Medicare. With the repeal of the act, the percentage covered by Medicare went back down to about 2 percent in 1990.

10. At Crescent, 85 percent were incontinent during my research, compared to 52 percent of the nation's nursing home residents in 1985 (Hing 1989). Sixty percent of Crescent residents needed assistance to eat at all (including 9 percent who were tube fed). At least another 15 percent needed constant prompting and encouragement to eat. Nationwide, in 1985, the figures are much lower: 39 percent of the nursing home population required assistance eating (ibid.). Only 14 percent of Crescent residents were ambulatory, including those who used a walker to get around.

11. This is similar to the national figure for 1985: 66 percent of nursing home residents were reported to have one mental disorder or more (Hing 1989).

12. In 1988, the turnover rate among patients at Crescent was about 30 percent. Fifty-one residents died in the home or hospital; 12 were discharged, either to a hospital, to the community, or to an institution offering a lower level of care. This turnover rate does not include residents who were readmitted after a hospital stay. When a resident of more than a month's standing is in the hospital for over 20 days, Medicaid stops paying for his or her bed. For these cases, when in official terminology the bedhold expires, the nursing home has an informal agreement with the nearby voluntary hospital; the hospital holds the resident until a bed at Crescent becomes available. In exchange, Crescent takes many of the hospital's patients.

13. According to the 1977 National Nursing Home Survey, 93 percent of nursing aides and orderlies in the United States were women (National Center for Health Statistics 1981).

14. Available figures on race and ethnicity for nursing aides refer to those

in all places of work, not just nursing homes. By 1987, 31 percent of nursing aides in the United States were black and 7 percent Hispanic, with the proportion steadily growing since the late 1970s (Quinlan 1988).

15. Why so many Caribbean immigrants are found in nursing aide work in New York City is a complex issue beyond the scope of this study. It is not simply a question of cheaper labor costs as New York nursing homes are largely unionized and offer relatively decent wages compared to other low-skilled work. As other studies of immigrants and the labor market show, network hiring and employer preferences are involved. Also, there is native blacks' desire to avoid traditional service jobs in which they have long been confined, as well as the opening up in recent years of opportunities for black Americans in white-collar jobs in the public sector (see Bailey and Waldinger 1991; Waldinger 1992; Waters 1992).

16. This includes those who were fired as well as those who left voluntarily. There is an extensive literature trying to explain the high national turnover rate among nursing aides, with analysts citing poor pay, lack of proper job orientation and adequate training, size of facility, staff characteristics such as age and educational level, and management style (see, e.g., Halbur 1982; Halbur and Fears 1986; Knapp and Harissis 1981; Schwartz 1974; Stryker 1981; Wallace and Brubaker 1982; and Waxman, Carner, and Berkenstock 1984).

17. Workers receive the maximum pension after 25 years.

18. Aides also receive a uniform and transportation allowance, totaling $4.50 a week when I did my research, and one free hot meal provided by the nursing home.

19. Similarly, Grau and her colleagues (1991) found that aides in the two New York City nursing homes they studied tended to be veteran workers, having been employed on average 11.3 years in their respective facilities.

20. See Diamond (1992: 13–24) for a description of the training program he attended, in Chicago, to become a certified nursing aide.

21. In January 1990, one aide at the Crescent Nursing Home (on the night shift) was accepted into the Ladders in Nursing Careers (LINC) program sponsored by the Greater New York Hospital Association. Her tuition was covered by the association; Crescent paid her a full salary though she only worked part-time (and went to school part-time). She owes Crescent a service payback of 18 months of full-time LPN work for every year of education she receives. Two LPNs at Crescent were also accepted into the LINC program to train to become RNs. Tuition scholarships are also available through the union for aides getting LPN training.

22. Two other nurses, one LPN and one RN, were Hispanic whites.

23. The shortages of the 1980s have eased, although there is still a demand for nurses in New York City.

24. Of the 18 top administrators and department heads, 5 were people of color when I did my research: the directors of admissions (black American) and food services (black American); nursing (Jamaican) and housekeeping (Dominican); and social services (Filipino). (When I arrived, the director of social services was white, but he was demoted and replaced by a Filipino colleague.) The 13 whites were administrator; assistant and associate adminis-

trators; and directors of activities, finance, development, medicine, physical therapy, occupational therapy, maintenance, volunteer services, systems management, and unit management services. As for gender, men did not dominate at the top: half of the top administrative and department heads, including a powerful associate administrator and the head of the primarily male food services department, were women.

3: Patients: Pressures, Frustrations, and Satisfactions

1. The labels given to aides' behavior toward patients inevitably reflect my own evaluations, yet there is good reason to believe that most outside observers would accept these characterizations in terms of the consequences for patients.

2. The 577 respondents were randomly selected from 57 New Hampshire nursing homes. Sixty-one percent were nursing aides, 20 percent LPNs, and 19 percent RNs.

3. Likewise, in his ethnography of a small, nonprofit nursing home in upstate New York, Savishinsky (1991) describes most staff, including aides, as conscientious about their work and only rarely treating patients improperly. He speaks of mistreatment of patients as "episodic, not systematic, in nature" (251).

4. Because the overwhelming majority of Crescent patients were non-Hispanic whites, I only mention ethnicity and/or race for the black and Hispanic patients I refer to by name.

5. This was not because she had another job. At Crescent, hardly any of the 35 on-staff day shift workers held other jobs, and it was unusual to do a double shift. This is different from what Diamond (1992) reports for the Chicago nursing homes he studied, where wages were much lower than at Crescent, less than $5 an hour. There, many aides had to do extra work or double shifts or had two jobs. Most aides at Crescent were not the sole wage earners in their households. For many, income from spouses' jobs and sometimes contributions from grown children and rent went into the total household income (see chap. 6).

6. Oliver and Tureman (1988: 84) note that the top two sources of satisfaction reported by more than 100 nursing aides at an educational seminar led by Oliver were the "joy of helping and caring for residents" and "appreciation I receive from those I care for."

7. In contrast, Kayser-Jones (1990: 47) says that attendants at the California nursing home she studied did not care what patients wore or how they looked. One woman normally sat in a wheelchair clad in a sweater and slip. (This would not have been tolerated by the Crescent administration.) Often, staff put bathrobes on backward to decrease the amount of work involved in changing incontinent patients.

8. Henderson (1987), an anthropologist who worked as an aide for 13

months, strikes a similar theme in speaking of his and his co-workers' need for kind words from residents, family members, and staff: "I found myself wishing for a little more understanding that we nurse aides were human, with feelings, trying to do a stressful job."

4: Institutional Demands: The "Iron Cage" of the Nursing Home

1. I rely heavily on Blau and Meyer (1987: 19–22) for the summary of Weber's definition of bureaucracy. Weber's ideal-type construct of bureaucracy was derived from abstracting the most characteristic bureaucratic aspects of all known organizations. It is a conceptual scheme to guide empirical research, not a description of any existing organization or an average of all organizations. It directs researchers to those aspects of organizations that must be examined to determine the extent of their bureaucratization (ibid., 25).

2. For an analysis of some unintended, negative consequences of government regulations for the evaluation and treatment of illnesses by nurses and physicians in nursing homes, see Wiener and Kayser-Jones's (1989) article, aptly subtitled "Accountability Gone Amok."

3. The cases presented in Kane and Caplan (1990) offer fascinating examples of ethical conflicts that arise in nursing homes, analyzed from the perspective of philosophers and ethicists. The cases show that residents' desire for autonomy often conflicts with the value of maintaining and enhancing their well-being, the interests of other residents, and the institution's concerns for safety, efficiency, and legal liability for injuries.

4. The inspection I witnessed had, as one of my favorite residents observed, elements of seriocomedy. Mr. Stone, a former high school teacher, a witty intellectual, and an acute observer of the nursing home's foibles, told me that the nurse who had been giving him medications for months would not even greet him before looking at his armband. (Officially, nurses must check armbands before giving medications to ensure they have the right patient.) Only after she looked at the armband did she say, "Hello, Mr. Stone," and go about her treatments. Thinking this was ridiculous, since the nurse obviously knew him well, he kidded her, saying, "I'm not Stone, I'm Schwartz [his roommate's name]. And you know, for a moment, an expression of doubt came across her face, and she thought she might have been treating the wrong person all this time."

5: Supervisors and the Nursing Hierarchy

1. In their study of two West Coast proprietary nursing homes, Wiener and Kayser-Jones (1989) also note aides' concern with culpability. One aide

they interviewed said, "I report every scratch. If I don't and the next shift does, I'm in trouble." Another said that she informed more than one nurse if a new symptom developed so she would not be blamed for causing it.

2. See Bowers and Becker (1992) on strategies for cutting corners among nursing aides in several midwestern homes they studied.

3. This closeness extended to socializing outside the nursing home, even across ethnic lines. The two Jamaican women were best friends at work and close off the job as well; the two black Americans frequently telephoned and saw each other outside of work. All four, however, invited each other to special parties and events like weddings and occasionally spoke on the telephone as well.

6: Family Ties

1. On the day shift, there were also family ties that did not involve nursing aides. A practical nurse had a daughter working as an administrative assistant; a young man in the housekeeping department got his job through his mother, an evening shift nursing aide. Savishinsky (1991: 178) also notes the use of kin ties for obtaining jobs in the nursing home he studied.

2. Wright (1988: 817) also suggests that infantilizing behavior may be an expression of caring, of giving a visual sign of having bathed and dressed a patient. Diamond (1992: 138) found that nursing aides often used the term "baby" to create fictive family roles and that it soothed some patients.

3. Two-thirds of the day shift aides on staff had school-aged children or grandchildren at home with them.

4. Protestant, as well as Catholic, aides send their children to Catholic schools. This is a common pattern in New York City, where about a quarter of the Catholic school student body is non-Catholic. Nearly all of the city's Catholic school students are from minority groups (Putka 1991).

5. In a study of 42 female staff members (including 26 nursing aides) in an intermediate care facility, Duffy and her associates (n.d.) found that nearly three-fourths said that residents' family members added to their stress.

7: Work Culture in the Nursing Home

1. In another kind of service work, family planning counseling, Joffe (1986) sees anticlient humor and other distancing devices as providing relief and some sense of dignity in a job that requires much selflessness. The activities she describes which distanced the counselors from clients did not, however, involve insults or jokes in front of clients, as in the nursing home context.

2. One exception was a couple of older aides who had trouble with taxing

physical tasks and were slow workers. Although they asked for help more often than they gave it, younger colleagues did not refuse, out of sympathy for the older women's difficulties and deference to their age.

3. Studies of several state mental institutions, carried out in the 1950s, emphasize the overwhelming negative effects of ward attendants' informal organization for patients. In one case, attendants developed a system whereby they rewarded some patients with privileges and punished others in brutal ways. Attendants who did not conform were reported and transferred to a less desirable ward (Belknap 1956). In another state mental hospital, informal practices among attendants stalemated a program of reform to improve patient care. The work culture perpetuated abusive behavior, including ridicule and customs that blocked patients from seeing the medical staff (Scheff 1961).

Whether this is still the case is unclear. In a California state mental hospital in the 1980s, the psychiatric technicians who provided most of the caregiving, unlike attendants of the past, had some formal training in psychiatric nursing, and many chose their careers because of concern for the mentally retarded. In contrast to earlier studies, Lundgren and Browner (1990) portray psychiatric technicians in consistently glowing terms: they treated residents with sympathy, love, and respect and allied themselves with residents against institutional policies they felt retarded the delivery of good care. Indeed, Lundgren and Browner see oppositional aspects of psychiatric technicians' work culture as nothing but positive for residents as well as workers, although surely some of the work culture strategies they mention, such as overlooking and covering up for workers who slacked off, abused residents, or came in late and telling jokes at residents' expense (within their hearing), had harmful effects.

4. Domestics who clean houses do not bear the same burden either when they struggle to resist employers' control and try to restructure the work process. When they develop routines to reduce the number of tasks or deliberately withhold information about cleaning supplies (Romero 1992), the result is a less clean house for a well-off, possibly irritated, employer. Obviously, this is much different for nursing aides, whose behavior can reduce the quality of care offered to frail, elderly patients.

5. Remember that service workers are almost as numerous as residents—some 140 service workers (including aides in the replacement pool) to 200 residents.

6. By the same token, recall from an earlier chapter how the director of nursing's race and ethnicity, black and Jamaican, in combination with her leadership style and displays of concern largely exempted her from aides' antagonism, despite her administrative position.

7. As laid out in the union contract, disciplinary actions follow set procedures. First comes a counseling conference. The next two steps are first and second written warnings, each preceded by notification to the union delegate. Then comes suspension and, finally, termination. The four steps preceding termination must take place within a relatively short period, say, 6 months, to lead to termination. In 1988, the administration issued 18 warnings and 1 suspension, most for lateness and absenteeism. Other grounds for the warn-

ings: argument, work performance, failure to follow the nursing care plan, not reporting an accident/incident, and inappropriate behavior to a nursing supervisor. During my fieldwork, one aide left before she was terminated (for consistent absenteeism), and the administration was building cases against another two aides.

8. At the time of the party, all but 4 of the 18 top administrators and department heads were white, as were most professionals outside of nursing.

8: Conclusion: Caregiving Dilemmas

1. In 1990, according to the Bureau of Labor Statistics, there were 595,000 nursing aides in nursing and personal care facilities; by 2005, the number is projected to be 942,000 (U.S. Department of Labor, Bureau of Labor Statistics, "National Industry-Occupational Matrix, 1990–2005").

2. For a beginning attempt in this direction see Watson and Maxwell's (1977) comparison of staff-resident relations at a Jewish and a black home for the elderly, in both of which cases nursing personnel were mostly black.

3. What distinguishes human service organizations is that people are their "raw material." The core activities of the organization are structured to process, sustain, or change people who come under its jurisdiction (Hasenfeld 1983, 1992). When I discuss people workers in human service organizations in this section, I am referring to nonprofessional workers rather than professionals or semiprofessionals like social workers or nurses.

4. Kayser-Jones (1990: 171) argues that the enforcement of state regulations has taken on such an enormous importance in this country that in many nursing homes, the goal becomes meeting, or appearing to meet, regulations rather than providing care. In her view, regulations mask the real problem, which is lack of professional responsibility for care. "An annual visit by a state inspection team," she writes, "will not ensure a high standard of care. This will only be achieved when there are an adequate number of knowledgeable, responsible professionals in the nursing home, planning, implementing, and monitoring care on a day-to-day basis." In fact, the Crescent Nursing Home has gone a good way toward solving the problems she mentions, with its permanent staff of excellent physicians, a first-rate gerontological nurse practitioner, and other professionals on staff. This study has identified other problems, for nonprofessional workers, that stem from a focus on meeting state regulations.

References

Abel, Emily, and Margaret Nelson. 1990. "Circles of Care: An Introductory Essay." In Emily Abel and Margaret Nelson, eds., *Circles of Care: Work and Identity in Women's Lives.* Albany: SUNY Press.

Aroskar, Mila, Ene K. Urv-Wong, and Rosalie Kane. 1990. "Building an Effective Caregiving Staff." In Rosalie Kane and Arthur Caplan, eds., *Everyday Ethics: Resolving Dilemmas in Nursing Home Life.* New York: Springer.

Ashley, JoAnn. 1976. *Hospitals, Paternalism, and the Role of the Nurse.* New York: Teachers College Press.

Bailey, Thomas, and Roger Waldinger. 1991. "The Changing Ethnic/Racial Division of Labor." In John Mollenkopf and Manuel Castells, eds., *Dual City: Restructuring New York.* New York: Russell Sage Foundation.

Belknap, Ivan. 1956. *Human Problems of a State Mental Hospital.* New York: McGraw Hill.

Bendix, Reinhard. 1960. *Max Weber: An Intellectual Portrait.* New York: Anchor Books.

Benson, Susan Porter. 1986. *Counter Cultures: Saleswomen, Managers, and Customers in American Department Stores, 1890–1940.* Urbana: University of Illinois Press.

Bishop, Katherine. 1989. "Studies Find Drugs Still Overused to Control Nursing Home Elderly." *New York Times,* March 13.

Blau, Peter, and Marshall Meyer. 1987. *Bureaucracy in Modern Society.* 3d ed. New York: Random House.

Bonnett, Aubrey. 1980. "An Examination of Rotating Credit Associations among Black West Indian Immigrants in Brooklyn." In R. S. Bryce-Laporte, ed., *Sourcebook on the New Immigration.* New Brunswick, N.J.: Transaction Books.

Bookman, Ann. 1988. "Unionization in an Electronics Factory: The Interplay of Gender, Ethnicity, and Class." In Ann Bookman and Sandra Morgen, eds., *Women and the Politics of Empowerment.* Philadelphia: Temple University Press.

Bould, Sally, Beverly Sanborn, and Laura Reif. 1989. *Eighty-Five Plus: The Oldest Old.* Belmont, Calif.: Wadsworth.

Bowers, Barbara. 1990. "Family Perceptions of Care in a Nursing Home." In Emily Abel and Margaret Nelson, eds., *Circles of Care.* Albany: SUNY Press.

Bowers, Barbara, and Marion Becker. 1989. "The Work World of Nursing Assistants in Long-Term Care." Paper presented at Gerontological Society of America meetings, Minneapolis.

———. 1992. "Nurse's Aides in Nursing Homes: The Relationship Between Organization and Quality." *The Gerontologist* 32: 360–366.

Brannon, Diane, Andrea Streit, and Michael Smyer. 1992. "The Psychosocial Quality of Nursing Home Work." *Journal of Aging and Health* 4: 369–389.

Burawoy, Michael. 1979. *Manufacturing Consent: Changes in the Labor Process under Monopoly Capitalism.* Chicago: University of Chicago Press.

Burbridge, Lynn. 1993. "The Labor Market for Home Care Workers: Demand, Supply, and Institutional Barriers." *The Gerontologist* 33: 41–46.

Cantor, Marjorie, and Elaine Chichin. 1990. *Stress and Strain among Homecare Workers of the Frail Elderly.* New York: Brookdale Research Institute on Aging, Fordham University.

Chandler, Jane, John Rachal, and Richard Kazelskis. 1986. "Attitudes of Long-Term Care Personnel Toward the Elderly." *The Gerontologist* 26: 551–555.

Chappell, Neena L., and Mark Novak. 1992. "The Role of Support in Alleviating Stress among Nursing Assistants." *The Gerontologist* 32: 351–359.

Coleman, Barbara. 1991. *The Nursing Home Reform Act of 1987: Provisions, Policy, Prospects.* Boston: University of Massachusetts, Gerontology Institute.

Cooper, Patricia. 1987. *Once a Cigar Maker: Men, Women, and Work Culture in American Cigar Factories, 1900–1919.* Urbana: University of Illinois Press.

Costello, Cynthia B. 1988. "Women Workers and Collective Action: A Case Study from the Insurance Industry." In Ann Bookman and Sandra Morgen, eds., *Women and the Politics of Empowerment.* Philadelphia: Temple University Press.

Diamond, Timothy. 1988. "Social Policy and Everyday Life in Nursing Homes." In Anne Statham, Eleanor Miller, and Hans Mauksch, eds., *The Worth of Women's Work.* Albany: SUNY Press.

———. 1990. "Nursing Homes as Trouble." In Emily Abel and Margaret Nelson, eds., *Circles of Care.* Albany: SUNY Press.

———. 1992. *Making Gray Gold: Narratives of Nursing Home Care.* Chicago: University of Chicago Press.

di Leonardo, Micaela. 1985. "Women's Work, Work Culture, and Consciousness." *Feminist Studies* 11: 491–496.

Duffy, JoAnn, Michael Duffy, Christopher Robinson, and Donald Barker.

N.d. "Family Linkage to Stress among Nursing Home Staff." Unpublished paper.

Eustis, Nancy, and Lucy Rose Fischer. 1991. "Relationships Between Home Care Clients and Their Workers: Implications for Quality Care." *The Gerontologist* 31: 447–456.

Eustis, Nancy, Lucy Rose Fischer, and Rosalie Kane. 1991. "Paraprofessional Home Care Workers and Quality of Care." Paper presented at the National Invitational Conference on Home Care Personnel Issues, Washington, D.C.

Feder, Barnaby. 1988. "What Ails a Nursing Home Empire." *New York Times,* December 11 (sec. 3, Business).

Feldman, Penny Hollander. 1993. "Work Life Improvements for Home Care Workers: Impact and Feasibility." *The Gerontologist* 33: 47–54.

Feldman, Penny Hollander, with Alice Sapienza and Nancy Kane. 1990. *Who Cares for Them: Workers in the Home Care Industry.* Westport: Greenwood Press.

Fischer, Lucy Rose, and Nancy Eustis. 1988. "DRGs and Family Care for the Elderly." *The Gerontologist* 28: 383–390.

Fisher, Ian. 1993. "With Care, Nursing Home Bridges Racial Gulf." *New York Times,* January 12.

Foner, Nancy. 1973. *Status and Power in Rural Jamaica.* New York: Teachers College Press.

———. 1978. *Jamaica Farewell: Jamaican Migrants in London.* Berkeley and Los Angeles: University of California Press.

Foner, Nancy, ed. 1987. *New Immigrants in New York.* New York: Columbia University Press.

Fontana, Andrea. 1977. *The Last Frontier.* Beverly Hills, Calif.: Sage.

Freeman, Iris C. 1990. "Developing Systems that Promote Autonomy: Policy Considerations." In Rosalie Kane and Arthur Caplan, eds., *Everyday Ethics: Resolving Dilemmas in Nursing Home Life.* New York: Springer.

Freeman, Iris C., and Bruce Vladeck. 1989. "The Nursing Home Conundrum." In Carl Eisdorfer, David Kessler, and Abby Spector, eds., *Caring for the Elderly.* Baltimore: Johns Hopkins University Press.

French, Howard. 1989. "Nursing Shortage, Wages and Tasks Grow." *New York Times,* December 4.

Geertz, Clifford. 1988. *Works and Lives.* Stanford: Stanford University Press.

Gerth, Hans, and C. Wright Mills. 1958. *From Max Weber: Essays in Sociology.* New York: Oxford University Press.

Giddens, Anthony. 1971. *Capitalism and Modern Social Theory.* Cambridge: Cambridge University Press.

Gilliland, Nancy, and Anne Brunton. 1984. "Nurses' Typification of Nursing Home Patients." *Ageing and Society* 4: 45–67.

Gluckman, Max. 1956. *Custom and Conflict in Africa.* Oxford: Basil Blackwell.

Goffman, Erving. 1961. *Asylums.* New York: Doubleday.

Grau, Lois, Barbara Chandler, Brenda Burton, and Doreen Kolditz. 1991. "Institutional Loyalty and Job Satisfaction among Nursing Aides in Nursing Homes." *Journal of Aging and Health* 3: 47–65.

Greene, Vernon L., and Deborah Monahan. 1982. "The Impact of Visitation on Patient Well-Being in Nursing Homes." *The Gerontologist* 22: 418–423.

Grenier, Guillermo, and Alex Stepick. 1992. "On Machines and Bureaucracy: Controlling Ethnic Interaction in Miami's Apparel and Construction Industries." In Louise Lamphere, ed., *Structuring Diversity: Ethnographic Perspectives on the New Immigration*. Chicago: University of Chicago Press.

Gubrium, Jaber F. 1975. *Living and Dying at Murray Manor*. New York: St. Martin's Press.

Halbur, Bernice. 1982. *Turnover among Nursing Personnel in Nursing Homes*. Ann Arbor: UMI Research Press.

Halbur, Bernice, and Neil Fears. 1986. "Nursing Personnel Turnover Rates Turned Over: Potential Positive Effects on Resident Outcomes in Nursing Homes." *The Gerontologist* 26: 70–77.

Halle, David. 1984. *America's Working Man*. Chicago: University of Chicago Press.

Handschu, S. S. 1973. "Profile of the Nurse's Aide." *The Gerontologist* 13: 315–317.

Hasenfeld, Yeheskel. 1983. *Human Service Organizations*. Englewood Cliffs, N.J.: Prentice-Hall.

———. 1992. "The Nature of Human Service Organizations." In Yeheskel Hasenfeld, ed., *Human Services as Complex Organizations*. Newbury Park, Calif.: Sage.

Heine, Christine A. 1986. "Burnout among Nursing Home Personnel." *Journal of Gerontological Nursing* 12: 14–18.

Henderson, J. Neil. 1987. "When a Professor Turns Nurse Aide." *Provider* 13: 8–12.

———. 1981. "Nursing Home Housekeepers: Indigenous Agents of Psychosocial Support." *Human Organization* 40: 300–305.

Hing, Esther. 1989. *Nursing Home Utilization by Current Residents: United States, 1985*. Hyattsville, Md.: National Center for Health Statistics.

Hochschild, Arlie. 1983. *The Managed Heart: Commercialization of Human Feeling*. Berkeley, Los Angeles, and London: University of California Press.

———. 1989. *The Second Shift: Inside the Two-Job Marriage*. New York: Viking.

Hooyman, Nancy, and Wendy Lustbader. 1986. *Taking Care: Supporting Older People and their Families*. New York: Free Press.

Institute of Medicine. 1986. *Improving the Quality of Care in Nursing Homes*. Washington, D.C.: National Academy Press.

Jayawardena, Chandra. 1963. *Conflict and Solidarity in a Guianese Plantation*. London: Athlone Press.

Joffe, Carole. 1986. *Regulation of Sexuality: Experiences of Family Planning Workers*. Philadelphia: Temple University Press.

Johnson, Colleen, and Leslie Grant. 1985. *The Nursing Home in American Society*. Baltimore: Johns Hopkins University Press.

Kahana, Eva, and H. Asuman Kiyak. 1984. "Attitudes and Behavior of Staff in Facilities for the Aged." *Research on Aging* 6: 395–416.

Kane, Robert L., and Rosalie A. Kane. 1978. "Care of the Aged: Old Problems in Need of New Solutions." *Science* 200: 913–919.

———. 1990. "Health Care for Older People: Organizational and Policy Issues." In Robert Binstock and Linda George, eds., *Handbook of Aging and the Social Sciences.* 3d ed. San Diego: Academic Press.

Kane, Rosalie A., and Arthur Caplan, eds. 1990. *Everyday Ethics: Resolving Dilemmas in Nursing Home Life.* New York: Springer.

Kanter, Rosabeth Moss. 1977. *Men and Women of the Corporation.* New York: Basic Books.

Kanter, Rosabeth Moss, and Barry Stein. 1979. "Making a Life at the Bottom." In Rosabeth Moss Kanter and Barry Stein, eds., *Life in Organizations.* New York: Basic Books.

Kayser-Jones, Jeanie Schmit. 1981. "A Comparison of Care in a Scottish and a United States Facility." *Geriatric Nursing* 2: 44–50.

———. 1983. "Social Exchange and Power in the Care of the Institutionalized Aged." *Human Organization* 42: 55–57.

———. 1990. *Old, Alone, and Neglected: Care of the Aged in Scotland and the United States.* Paperback ed. with epilogue. Berkeley, Los Angeles, and London: University of California Press.

Kemper, Peter, and Christopher Murtaugh. 1991. "Lifetime Use of Nursing Home Care." *New England Journal of Medicine* 324: 595–600.

Kjervik, Diane. 1990. "Beyond the Call of Duty: A Nurse's Aide Uses Her Judgment." In Rosalie A. Kane and Arthur Caplan, eds., *Everyday Ethics: Resolving Dilemmas in Nursing Home Life.* New York: Springer.

Knapp, Martin, and Kostas Harissis. 1981. "Staff Vacancies and Turnover in British Old People's Homes." *The Gerontologist* 21: 76–84.

Lamphere, Louise. 1985. "Bringing the Family to Work: Women's Culture on the Shop Floor." *Feminist Studies* 11: 519–540.

———. 1987. *From Working Daughters to Working Mothers.* Ithaca: Cornell University Press.

Lamphere, Louise, Patricia Zavella, and Felipe Gonzales. 1993. *Sunbelt Working Mothers: Reconciling Family and Factory.* Ithaca: Cornell University Press.

Lerea, L. Eliezer, and Barbara F. LiMauro. 1982. "Grief among Healthcare Workers: A Comparative Study." *Journal of Gerontology* 37: 604–608.

Light, Ivan. 1972. *Ethnic Enterprise in America.* Berkeley and Los Angeles: University of California Press.

Lundgren, Rebecka Inga, and Carole H. Browner. 1990. "Caring for the Institutionalized Mentally Retarded: Work Culture and Work-Based Social Support." In Emily Abel and Margaret Nelson, eds., *Circles of Care.* Albany: SUNY Press.

MacAdam, Margaret. 1993. "Home Care Reimbursement and Effects on Personnel." *The Gerontologist* 33: 55–63.

Mechanic, David. 1976. *The Growth of Bureaucratic Medicine: An Inquiry into the Dynamics of Patient Behavior and the Organization of Medical Care.* New York: Wiley.

———. 1989. *Painful Choices: Research and Essays on Health Care.* New Brunswick, N.J.: Transaction.

Melosh, Barbara. 1982. *"The Physician's Hand": Work Culture and Conflict in American Nursing*. Philadelphia: Temple University Press.

Merton, Robert K. 1957. "Bureaucratic Structure and Personality." In R. Merton, *Social Theory and Social Structure*. New York: Free Press.

Montgomery, David. 1979. *Workers' Control in America*. Cambridge: Cambridge University Press.

Morgen, Sandra. 1990. "Beyond the Double Day: Work and Family in Working-Class Women's Lives." *Feminist Studies* 16: 53–67.

National Center for Health Statistics. 1981. *Employees in Nursing Homes in the United States: 1977 National Nursing Home Survey*. Hyattsville, Md.: U.S. Department of Health and Human Services.

Oliver, David B., and Sally Tureman. 1988. *The Human Factor in Nursing Home Care*. New York: Haworth Press.

Ortner, Sherry. 1984. "Theory in Anthropology Since the Sixties." *Comparative Studies in Society and History* 26: 126–166.

Paules, Greta Foff. 1991. *Dishing It Out: Power and Resistance among Waitresses in a New Jersey Restaurant*. Philadelphia: Temple University Press.

Penner, Louis, Krista Ludenia, and Gayle Mead. 1984. "Staff Attitudes: Image or Reality?" *Journal of Gerontological Nursing* 10: 110–117.

Perrow, Charles. 1986. *Complex Organizations: A Critical Essay*. 3d ed. New York: Random House.

Pessar, Patricia. 1987. "The Dominicans: Women in the Household and the Garment Industry." In Nancy Foner, ed., *New Immigrants in New York*. New York: Columbia University Press.

Pillemer, Karl, and David Moore. 1989. "Abuse of Patients in Nursing Homes: Findings from a Survey of Staff." *The Gerontologist* 29: 314–320.

Pleck, Elizabeth. 1976. "Two Worlds in One." *Journal of Social History* 10: 178–195.

Portes, Alejandro, and Robert Bach. 1985. *Latin Journey: Cuban and Mexican Immigrants in the United States*. Berkeley, Los Angeles, and London: University of California Press.

Putka, Gary. 1991. "NY Archdiocese Begins Campaign to Save 140 Catholic Schools in the City." *Wall Street Journal*, January 30.

Quinlan, Alice. 1988. *Chronic Care Workers: Crisis among Paid Caregivers of the Elderly*. Washington, D.C.: Older Women's League.

Reeder, Sharon, and Hans Mauksch. 1979. "Nursing: Continuing Change." In Howard Freeman, Sol Levine, and Hans Mauksch, eds., *Handbook of Medical Sociology*. 3d ed. Englewood Cliffs, N.J.: Prentice-Hall.

Rhodes, Lorna A. 1991. *Emptying Beds: The Work of an Emergency Psychiatric Unit*. Berkeley, Los Angeles, and Oxford: University of California Press.

Roethlisberger, F. J., and William J. Dickson. 1939. *Management and the Worker*. Cambridge: Harvard University Press.

Romero, Mary. 1992. *Maid in the U.S.A.* New York: Routledge.

Roy, Donald. 1958. "'Banana Time': Job Satisfaction and Informal Interaction." *Human Organization* 18: 158–168.

Rubin, Allen, and Guy Shuttlesworth. 1983. "Engaging Families as Support Resources in Nursing Home Care: Ambiguity in the Subdivision of Tasks." *The Gerontologist* 23: 632–636.

Rudder, Cynthia. 1988. *Reimbursement and the Nursing Home Resident: Resource Utilization Groups.* New York: State of New York, Department of Health.

———. 1989. *Case Mix Reimbursement and the Nursing Home Resident in New York State.* New York: Nursing Home Coalition of New York State.

Sacks, Karen B. 1988. *Caring by the Hour: Women, Work and Organizing at Duke Medical Center.* Urbana: University of Illinois Press.

Savishinsky, Joel S. 1991. *The Ends of Time: Life and Work in a Nursing Home.* New York: Bergin and Garvey.

Scheff, Thomas J. 1961. "Control over Policy Attendants in a Mental Hospital." *Journal of Health and Human Behavior* 2: 93–105.

Schwartz, Arthur. 1974. "Staff Development and Morale Building in Nursing Homes." *The Gerontologist* 14: 50–53.

Schwartz, Arthur, and Mark Vogel. 1990. "Nursing Home Staff and Residents' Families Role Expectations." *The Gerontologist* 30: 49–53.

Schwartz, Howard, Peggy de Wolf, and James Skipper. 1987. "Gender, Professionalization, and Occupational Anomie: The Case of Nursing." In Howard Schwartz, ed., *Dominant Issues in Medical Sociology.* New York: Random House.

Shapiro-Perl, Nina. 1984. "Resistance Strategies: The Routine Struggle for Bread and Roses." In Karen B. Sacks and Dorothy Remy, eds., *My Troubles Are Going to Have Trouble with Me.* New Brunswick, N.J.: Rutgers University Press.

Sheridan, John E., John White, and Thomas J. Fairchild. 1992. "Ineffective Staff, Ineffective Supervision, or Ineffective Administration? Why Some Nursing Homes Fail to Provide Adequate Care." *The Gerontologist* 32: 334–341.

Shield, Renée Rose. 1988. *Uneasy Endings: Daily Life in an American Nursing Home.* Ithaca: Cornell University Press.

Short, Pamela Farley, Peter Kemper, Llewellyn Cornelius, and Daniel Walden. 1992. "Public and Private Responsibility for Financing Nursing-Home Care: The Effect of Medicaid Asset Spend-down." *Milbank Quarterly* 70: 277–298.

Smith, Kristen, and Vern Bengtson. 1979. "Positive Consequences of Institutionalization: Solidarity between Elderly Parents and Their Middle-Aged Children." *The Gerontologist* 19: 438–447.

Sperbeck, David J., and Susan K. Whitbourne. 1981. "Dependency in the Institutional Setting: A Behavioral Training Program for Geriatric Staff." *The Gerontologist* 21: 268–275.

Stannard, Charles. 1973. "Old Folks and Dirty Work: The Social Conditions for Patient Abuse in a Nursing Home." *Social Problems* 20: 329–342.

Stein, Leonard. 1967. "The Doctor-Nurse Game." *Archives of General Psychiatry* 16: 699–703.

Strahan, Genevieve. 1987. "Nursing Home Characteristics, Preliminary Data from the 1985 National Nursing Home Survey." *Advance Data From Vital and Health Statistics.* No. 131. Hyattsville, Md.: National Center for Health Statistics, Public Health Service.

Stryker, R. 1981. *How to Reduce Employee Turnover in Nursing Homes and Other Health Care Organizations*. Springfield, Ill.: Charles C. Thomas.

Tellis-Nayak, V. 1988. *Nursing Home Exemplars of Quality*. Springfield, Ill.: Charles C. Thomas.

Tellis-Nayak, V., and Mary Tellis-Nayak. 1989. "Quality of Care and the Burden of Two Cultures: When the World of the Nurse's Aide Enters the World of the Nursing Home." *The Gerontologist* 29: 307–313.

Tentler, Leslie Woodcock. 1979. *Wage-Earning Women: Industrial Work and Family Life in the United States, 1900–1930*. New York: Oxford University Press.

Ullmann, Steven G. 1987. "Ownership, Regulation, Quality Assessment and Performance in the Long-Term Health Care Industry." *The Gerontologist* 27: 233–239.

United Hospital Fund of New York. 1988. *Facilities for the Aging: How to Choose a Nursing Home*. New York: United Hospital Fund of New York.

United States Department of Labor. 1991. "National Industry-Occupational Matrix, 1990–2005," Bureau of Labor Statistics.

United States Senate Special Committee on Aging. 1991. *Aging America—Trends and Projections*. Washington, D.C.: U.S. Department of Health and Human Services.

Vesperi, Maria. 1983. "The Reluctant Consumer: Nursing Home Residents in the Post-Bergman Era." In Jay Sokolovsky, ed., *Growing Old in Different Societies*. Belmont, Calif.: Wadsworth.

Vladeck, Bruce. 1980. *Unloving Care: The Nursing Home Tragedy*. New York: Basic Books.

Waldinger, Roger. 1992. "Taking Care of the Guests: The Impact of Immigrants on Services—An Industry Case Study." *International Journal of Urban and Regional Research* 16: 97–113.

Wallace, Robert W., and Timothy H. Brubaker. 1982. "Biographical Factors Related to Employment Tenure: A Study of Nurse Aides in Nursing Homes." *Journal of Long-Term Care Administration* (Spring): 11–19.

Waters, Mary. 1992. "Hiring Practices and Racial and Ethnic Dynamics at American Food Services." Unpublished paper.

Watson, Wilbur H., and Robert Maxwell. 1977. *Human Aging and Dying*. New York: St. Martin's Press.

Waxman, Howard M., Erwin A. Carner, and Gale Berkenstock. 1984. "Job Turnover and Job Satisfaction among Nursing Home Aides." *The Gerontologist* 24: 503–509.

Weber, George. 1990. *Geriatric Nursing Assistants: An Annotated Bibliography with Models to Enhance Practice*. New York: Greenwood Press.

Weber, Max. 1958. *The Protestant Ethic and the Spirit of Capitalism*. New York: Charles Scribner's.

———. [1947] 1964. *The Theory of Social and Economic Organization*. New York: Free Press.

Westwood, Sallie. 1985. *All Day, Everyday: Factory and Family in the Making of Women's Lives*. Urbana: University of Illinois Press.

Wiener, Carolyn, and Jeanie Kayser-Jones. 1989. "Defensive Work in Nursing

Homes: Accountability Gone Amok." *Social Science and Medicine* 28: 37–44.

Wolff, Craig. 1987. "Nursing Homes Want Fewer of the Not-So-Ill." *New York Times*, August 28.

Wright, Lore. 1988. "A Reconceptualization of the 'Negative Staff Attitudes and Poor Care in Nursing Homes' Assumption." *The Gerontologist* 28: 813–820.

Zavella, Patricia. 1987. *Women's Work and Chicano Families.* Ithaca: Cornell University Press.

Index

Designer: U.C. Press Staff
Compositor: Prestige Typography
Text: 10/13 Galliard
Display: Galliard
Printer: Maple-Vail Book Manufacturing Group
Binder: Maple-Vail Book Manufacturing Group

PENSACOLA JUNIOR COLLEGE LIBRARY
3 5101 01005004 0

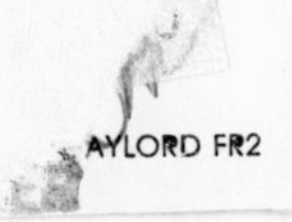
AYLORD FR2